# NOW ANL _ _

Julia Burton-Jones spent several years researching the issues of ageing and caring while working for the Jubilee Centre in Cambridge. Between 1990 and 1992 she initiated and ran a series of training seminars for churches, entitled 'Action for Family Carers', and she has recently been involved in setting up the Carers Christian Fellowship, a new group for carers. Her book *Caring for Carers* was published by Scripture Union in 1992, and she has since written another book, *Caring for your Elderly Parent*, published by Sheldon Press in 1996.

# NOW AND FOREVER

## Reflections on
## the Later Years of Life

JULIA BURTON-JONES

**TRIANGLE**

First published in Great Britain 1997
Triangle Books
Holy Trinity Church
Marylebone Road
London NW1 4DU

Biblical quotations are from the *New International Version*,
© 1973, 1978, 1984 by the International Bible Society.
Published by Hodder & Stoughton.

NOTE
Every effort has been made to trace the copyright holders
of material quoted here. Information on any omissions
should be sent to the publishers who will make full
acknowledgement in any future editions.

British Library Cataloguing-in-Publication Data
A catalogue record of this book is available
from the British Library

ISBN 0-281-04992-0

Typeset by Pioneer Associates, Perthshire
Printed in Great Britain by
Biddles Ltd, Guildford and King's Lynn

# Contents

*For Timothy and Helena*

# Acknowledgements

My thanks are extended to the many retired people who have given so freely of themselves in contributing to this book. I thank them for opening their hearts to me and to all those who want to find through reading this a better understanding of what it means to be older.

I am also grateful to my editor, Naomi Starkey. The inspiration for *Now and Forever* was hers and her advice throughout the process of completing it has been greatly valued. I have also relied heavily on the encouragement, not to mention practical assistance, of my husband, Simon. Finally, without the selfless support of my sisters, Lois, Helen and Claire-Lise it would not have been possible to reach the conclusion of this most challenging, though rewarding, piece of work whilst remaining in possession of my sanity!

# Introduction

This book is a celebration of old age. It does not belittle the suffering many people face in their later years, but it seeks to present retirement in all its rich variety of experience. Contributors to the book portray later life as being full of meaning and purpose, not the bit of life to be 'got through' when the real business of living is over. Many seem to have discovered the secret of living for each moment, of living with conviction and with a confidence that they know what matters to them more assuredly than ever before. Opportunities for growth are embraced willingly. The God who has been present, but sometimes elusive, since their early years has often become someone with whom they commune more naturally. There is a spirit of adventure, an appreciation of the freedom retirement brings, and a broader and deeper love for the whole of humanity.

If I speak with unmeasured enthusiasm about the scope for fulfilment and personal development in retirement, I make no apologies. I emphasize the positive aspects of ageing in order to counter the predominantly pessimistic assessments of later life which currently prevail in Western societies. The voices we hear speaking about ageing in the public domain are not the voices of older people. They are the voices of politicians spreading alarm over the rising cost of caring for very elderly people. They are the voices

of a culture which extols the virtues of being young. Even
the people who research the process of ageing have not
reached old age themselves in the majority of cases. A
whole host of so-called 'authorities' on ageing have denied
older people the opportunity to define for themselves the
nature of old age.

This book attempts to redress the balance a little by
turning to older people themselves for insights into the
meaning of later life. It does not pretend to offer a statisti-
cally sound analysis of ageing. It provides snapshots of
the lives of a group of individuals whose experiences of life,
and so also of retirement, have varied greatly. The one
thing they each have in common is an allegiance to the
Christian faith. In other ways they are very different. They
differ in social and occupational backgrounds and in their
experiences of family life, and they range in age from the
newly retired through to a centenarian.

A piece of research to which I turn often is a survey
undertaken by British Gas in 1991. This survey made a
special contribution to the debate on ageing because it
obtained its data 'from the horse's mouth', asking older
people themselves how they felt about retirement. It gave
a refreshingly new perspective. For example, it asked older
people what they preferred to be called, and found, unexpectedly, that they did not like being called 'elderly',
'pensioners' or 'older people'. Instead they liked the titles
'retired' or 'senior citizen'.

The British Gas survey was heartening in that it found
that most older people were happy with their lives. The
majority were not ill, or lonely, or overdependent on other
people. It is also the aim of this book to present knowledge
on ageing which is derived from people who have actually
experienced later life.

One factor fuelling concern over caring for the elderly
population is the increase in the population in the numbers
of those aged over eighty. In the Policy Studies Institute
report, *Britain in 2010* (1991), figures show that, whilst

the numbers aged 65-79 will remain roughly the same between 1990 and 2010, there will be a 26 per cent increase in the over-eighties. This is on top of a 73 per cent increase in this age group between 1970 and 1990. It is feared that the taxes paid by the working population will be insufficient to cover the cost of caring for the very elderly when they become frail. Some disagree with the alarmist view of demography which this view represents (the House of Commons Health Committee, for instance, reported in August 1996 that it anticipated no crisis in the National Health Service as a result of our ageing population). Nevertheless, scare-mongering over future care costs has exerted a negative influence on responses to rising numbers of very elderly people in our society.

It would be nice if for once, instead of presenting older people as a potential burden to society, media reports were to stress the valuable contribution so many retired people are making to their local communities. The older population give far more than they receive, and even those who do depend on others for support can continue to play a vital role as members of their families and neighbourhoods.

It is puzzling that so much credence is given to presentations of later life as a parasitic stage of existence. It is also strange that the adulation of youth is so rarely questioned. Even older people feel they have value only when they are able to mimic those younger than themselves. In other cultures age is revered and respected; being older is something to cherish, a time of life to anticipate with pleasure. Yet in the Bible there is plenty of positive comment on later life, which Christians could offer as a critique of contemporary philosophies of ageing. The Bible portrays age as something to be honoured, as a time of wisdom and spiritual maturity.

Mary Thomas, who writes in chapter 2, expresses frustration over the unwillingness of younger people to accept that older people are not members of an alien race. She wishes they could recognize their future selves in the older

people they meet. There is an interesting psychological
process at work, it seems. Younger people prefer to pretend
that ageing will never happen to them. By treating older
people as a strange species they can continue to act as if
they will never be old themselves. In fact retirement will
come to most of us and it may last many years. It is not
like any other stage of life: if we are to enjoy it to the full,
we must plan for it. And yet there is no formal process of
preparation, no 'rite of passage' as the anthropologists
would call it, which governs retirement. When we marry
we spend time and thought in achieving readiness for the
upheaval involved. There is the gradual build-up to the day
itself. Then there is the ritual of the marriage ceremony
which makes us aware of the implications of the step we are
taking. Retirement, on the other hand, steals up on us
quietly. From an absorption in the demands of our working lives we move to a phase of existence where we must
discover for ourselves daily structure and activity.

Retirement is too lengthy to be frittered away in idle
entertainment. For the Christian there is the imperative to
be usefully employed in the work of the kingdom of God,
perhaps through new areas of service and ministry. There
is the need to find meaning and motivation. Certainly
there is scope for growing towards maturity in the faith.
Throughout the vicissitudes of later life, its pain and its
exhilaration, we can learn more of God's purposes. There
is no excuse for taking a rest from the call to discipleship.

It is hoped that this book will help readers to understand
the new way of life which retirement brings. It may encourage the not-yet-retired to think ahead and visualize ways in
which their later years could be filled with worthwhile
activity. It may enable them to adjust their expectations.
The older people whose lives are featured through the
pages of this book are remarkably frank in their accounts
of their experiences. They admit to failings and rejoice
over accomplishments. They each have a story of God's
faithfulness to tell.

It is wise to remember, however, that the retired people who appear here do not form a cross-section of British pensioners. They were not randomly selected! They are all Christians and quite a number have worked in full-time Christian ministry. Many have had exceptional lives, achieving the highest honours in their chosen careers and attaining nationwide recognition. Few have known low income in retirement, although in actual fact pensioners form a large proportion of Britain's poor. The benefits of an illustrious working life and a comfortable standard of living considerably enhance the circumstances of later life. Several contributors, for example, have continued to pursue professional interests well into retirement. Such continuity is a blessing not easily achieved in all areas of work.

In a sense, people who are willing to write about retirement are likely to be those for whom it is a good experience. They are also perhaps individuals who possess the ability and inclination to reflect on their lives. There were others who were invited to contribute but declined for a variety of reasons. Some were not in a position to be involved because their time was already filled to capacity. This was encouraging to hear and conveyed the impression of motivation and fulfilment. Others said they were not really retired in that they intended to continue with their life's work to their dying day, God willing. But there were also others for whom the idea of writing about their own ageing seemed a disturbing prospect. Several replied to the effect that they did not 'feel old', though they clearly were advanced in years. It was almost as if they were trying to escape the reality of their age, as if admitting being old would be to embrace a status of little consequence. I wondered if their response would have been different had they been asked to write a chapter for a book on Christian leadership!

I am very grateful to each of the people who have willingly associated themselves with this book on ageing.

Some of them have many calls on their time, and part of their reason for taking the trouble to put their thoughts about retirement into words has been the desire to help others view it more accurately and more positively. Many have welcomed the opportunity to bear witness to God's loving influence upon their lives.

Much of the material contained in the book, whether poetry or prose, is original writing which has appeared nowhere else. Some of it has featured elsewhere, as indicated, and is reproduced with the permission of the author. Mostly contributors have written their own accounts, but in some cases I have drawn together the thoughts and feelings they have expressed in lengthy and rewarding conversations. I have also included occasional paragraphs from other books which deal with the issue of ageing. Some of the people who were asked to write for the book chose to address several of the chapter topics. Others wrote more generally and I have placed their pieces in the chapters where they seemed most readily to fit.

The scope of *Now and Forever* is considerable. It touches on most issues which have a bearing on retirement. My hope is that it conveys an impression of retirement as a time of tremendous opportunity, deep fulfilment and bracing challenge. My sincere wish is that reading this book will cause people who have harboured anxieties about being older to look forward to the later stages of their life, and to expect to find there the fulfilment of each preceding era.

# 1

# Forging a New Role

Retirement is something we have come to take for granted as a natural stage in our lives. Yet it is actually a relatively new phenomenon. Until the twentieth century older people did not withdraw from work when they reached a certain age. Only as we began to live longer did we think about ways of occupying people who were older.

It is a big step to go from being a full-time worker one day to being completely free of the obligations of work the next. For this reason many firms now offer their employees pre-retirement preparation to help them think ahead and plan for the future. This works best of all when participants are asked to take a broad view and think about how to use their time and freedom, rather than focusing only on the practicalities of housing, income, investments and the like. But whether they are well prepared or not, the majority of older people feel positive about retirement. They relish the thought of being free to choose how to spend their time after years of being governed by the demands of work.

The question which emerges, however, as Pam Wyatt puts it in this chapter, is do we retire 'from' something, or do we retire 'to' a new role? Do senior citizens have special responsibilities, a unique contribution to make to society?

Talking to some pensioners you might easily conclude that they regard retirement as a time to rest after their years of paid work, an opportunity to enjoy leisure pursuits and

7

hobbies, to idle away the hours. They have 'done their bit', as it were, and believe that they can legitimately hand on their productive role to the next generation. You almost feel that obligations of any kind are unwelcome and intrusive. The British Gas survey uncovered something of this in the lifestyles of older people. They spent a lot of time watching TV and pottering in the garden, and surprisingly few people were involved in more outward-looking activities such as voluntary work.

It would be encouraging to think that we could develop more positive ideas about later life. Retirement could be viewed as a time of opportunity in which to pursue new areas of work and service. In place of idleness, there would be constructive activity designed to build community and family.

The retired people who have contributed to this chapter have exercised great initiative in planning their lives as senior citizens. Many are fortunate to have spent their working lives in careers they can carry over into retirement; the blessing of continuity this offers is not to be underestimated. There is a sense also, however, in which the centrality of faith in the lives of these older people acts as a driving force and provides the impetus to seek purposeful, often altruistic activity. For many, retirement has given them the chance to experience a fresh 'calling' and to seek new areas for service and ministry.

## PAM WYATT

When I was in my early fifties I deliberately pushed any thought of retirement to the back of my mind. I loved my job, finding it tremendously stimulating and rewarding, and the thought of leaving it in around ten years' time filled me with anxiety.

Quite unexpectedly, I was faced with an operation which entailed three months' convalescence at home. Although I had no fears about the operation itself, I wondered how

I would cope with all that time on my hands, especially as I would be unable to drive or walk any distance. I had lived on my own for a number of years, so I would have to rely on other people to provide company and do shopping for me. Not a happy thought for someone who prided herself on her independence, and perhaps a foretaste of how things would be in old age! Retirement for me at that time meant a giving up, and certainly not a gaining, and now I was to experience three months of boredom which would prove how right I was to fear the future.

To my great surprise, it turned out to be one of the most rewarding periods of my life, and a time when God taught me some important lessons about myself and my relationship with him. This was particularly necessary in regard to trust (or lack of it) and pride (how would they manage without me at work). I found that I had unlimited time to read, think and pray without interruption. Silence became a joy, and solitude a lasting need in my life, rather than something to be feared.

However, I was still thinking of the future as retiring *from* rather than retiring *to*. But God, who had already surprised me by showing me the joy of being 'beside quiet waters', had more in store for me and took me into a new relationship and the blessing of a second marriage.

My husband and I both believed that God had brought us together for more than 'the mutual society, help and comfort that one ought to have of the other', although that was certainly an important part of it. For some time, my husband had been hoping for an early retirement so that he could give more time to working for the Lord. We wondered if this was now the right time to change direction in this way. Although people at his place of work were being asked to consider early retirement, his application was turned down and we took the decision to see if perhaps God was calling me to a new way of life instead.

This time I had no regrets about leaving a job which gave me so much personal satisfaction. It took some time to discover how God wanted to use me, and I had to abandon some ideas of my own on the way. Eventually it became clear that I was being led into a 'ministry of availability' and that is what has engaged my time and energy for some years now. It has involved teaching, listening, counselling, befriending, helping in practical ways, and praying with people in many different situations, all of which I had been trained for many years ago.

What happened to all that spare time I thought I would have? There has not been much of that, but there has been enough to enjoy activities I had not had sufficient time for before. Retirement has proved to be a beginning, not an end; a time to look forward with anticipation to the future, rather than looking back with regret.

## PROFESSOR BARONESS McFARLANE OF LLANDAFF

I came to retirement suddenly and with inadequate planning. When I was appointed to the first Chair of Nursing in an English university, my letter of appointment was until the September following my sixty-seventh birthday. Retirement age in the university was equal for men and women! I was so occupied with the challenges of new developments in my department that I gave little thought to my own future, expecting to reach retirement in 1993. It never crossed my mind to take early retirement. I think I almost saw myself as indispensable! Suitably qualified academics in my discipline were still rare. But then a colleague of about the same age told me that she had explored the terms of the early retirement scheme and decided that she would go. Out of curiosity I asked for particulars of how early retirement would affect me. I found that if I worked until I was sixty-seven, I would be no better off financially. I recognized that I was tired, and in the space of a week (the time that was left before applications had to be in) I made the decision to go at the end of the academic year. That is not ideal. I would advise anyone else to plan carefully in advance, but I have to admit that, with less than a full term left to work, I looked forward to the end of my working life at sixty-two with some excitement, if foreboding! I have now been retired for eight years.

But life does not begin or end with retirement. It builds on the foundation of life experiences that have gone before, and stretches out into a future which seeks to use those experiences to look ahead creatively.

I read chemistry at university because that had been my best subject at school. But during my first year God drew me into a much closer relationship with him. There followed a process of waiting and listening to find out where he was leading me and this became a pattern in all the career changes of my life. I became convinced that I should follow a career in nursing. I then trained in midwifery and health visiting and eventually in nursing education.

Once in nursing education I was given wide-ranging experiences which led to my directing the first clinical nursing research project in this country, aimed at establishing criteria for measuring the quality of nursing care. At the same time I was building up my own academic credibility and eventually I became first a senior lecturer and then Professor of Nursing at the University of Manchester.

Because of its pioneering work, the department in Manchester became something of an international centre. I became personally involved in exploring the ethics and philosophy of nursing, attempting to identify the value system which underlies nursing practice. This was a marvellous opportunity to explore the way my faith related to my work.

Because I had retired in a hurry, the early days of retirement were spent taking stock and throwing out a challenge to God: 'You called me into nursing, now you will need to show me what you want me to do next. I need a second calling!' I remember surveying the rather nasty hole that I thought the absence of work would leave and praying, 'Please fill my life for you'. I am not sure that I envisaged how literally that might have been answered, because there have been times when I have had to stand back and say, 'Now what do I say no to?' I am still not very good at saying no and can easily become overloaded.

Many of the abilities that I developed in my working life have been used in different ways and for different organizations in my retirement. At first I taught mature students. It was nice to have continuing contact, but I felt it was right to put an end to this after a year. At the same time I decided to give up lecturing.

Teaching was a skill that had become very much a part of me. That seems to have been taken and used in other settings. Christian Viewpoint meetings are organized by Christian women. They aim to bring their friends together for coffee, lunch or supper and a speaker. I must have spoken at dozens of these meetings and find great fulfilment in sharing my faith with other women. Although I am not a Reader, I have a regular input into the preaching schedule of my local church. I find this a wonderful stimulation and challenge. I use my old skills of reading and researching a subject, but there is an added dimension in listening to the Holy Spirit and hearing what he wants to say to the congregation.

One of the skills I had to cultivate in academic life was committee work. In retirement I have been able to continue using these skills though often in different contexts. For five years I was a member of the General Synod of the Church of England. I am now serving on the Synod Review Group which gives me an opportunity to voice my concerns, and I have also served on the Hospital Chaplains' Council. But the work I have in retirement which is significantly different from that of most is in the House of Lords. In 1979, when I was offered a life peerage, I was concerned to be a follower of Christ in a place which has so many associations with power and glory. Since I have been there I have been glad that from time to time my nursing background, my experience in education and my Christian faith have been relevant to many of the topics under discussion. Very early on the Human Fertilization and Embryo Bill was under discussion. I have served on the Select Committee on Medical Ethics and two Select Committees on Research in the National Health Service and the Effects of NHS Reforms on Research. It is good to see my experience used in this way, although as I get further removed from day-to-day involvement, I have to work harder to make my contribution meaningful.

## PAUL TOURNIER

### A Second Career

The revaluation of old age and of the status of the retired person demands a far-reaching change in the attitude of the public. But it also depends on the initiative of retired people themselves, on the use they make of the freedom and time that retirement affords them . . . It is for us old people to build our own lives, lives that are worthwhile, interesting and worthy of respect, and so to arouse fresh hope in the young that they can look forward to a happy old age. It is for us to show that it is possible to live a life that is different from our working life, but quite as useful and satisfying . . . .

You have complained for so many years of being rushed, of not having enough time. Now that you have time, what use are you making of it? You feel you have been relegated, but is it not a fact that you allow yourself to be too easily relegated? Are you not conniving a little in your own relegation, through your passivity? People talk a little too much about leisure occupations, about hobbies. I invite you to have more ambition . . . I put forward this idea of a second

career in order to stimulate you, to arouse your imagi-
nation and zeal ... There is no lack of opportunities
for self-improvement in this world, even at an
advanced age. What is most often wrong is that people do not open their eyes to see the opportunities,
that they fail to grasp them, and do not have confidence enough to succeed.

From Paul Tournier's *Learning to Grow Old*
(English tr., SCM Press 1972).

## BISHOP JOHN TAYLOR AND HIS WIFE
## LINDA TAYLOR

### Bishop John

For someone like myself who has lived throughout my
career in the Church in tied accommodation, the first and
most difficult adjustment in retirement is the decision
about where one is to live. It is the first time in one's life
that there has been any real choice. No longer is it a
matter of deciding whether a particular job is the right
kind of challenge. Now one has to choose where one is
going to live out of all the houses and bungalows in the
whole country – and why be restricted to the UK, for that
matter? Money aside, and of course that is a prominent
factor influencing the selection, the choice is limitless.

We decided that a university town would have its attrac-
tions. We wanted to live somewhere where there was a
degree of culture, as well as some intellectual stimulus, be
it evening classes, concerts, lectures, a library ... That
was true for my wife as well as myself. I also wanted to be
within reach of a lively church that would not depend
upon me too much, and some top quality worship, as in a
cathedral or college chapel. Cambridge seemed to provide
the answer.

It was a good decision. We are deeply happy and feel
privileged to be here, not too far from old friends, within

easy reach of family without being on top of them, and with access to good motorways and transport. Evening visits to London are not impossible for less than £10 return fare.

Retirement so far has felt rather like an extended honeymoon. We have been able to do what we want, and do it together, in a way that has never been possible before. The first 'pleasure' was having the time to walk to the postbox with my own letters instead of dropping them in from the car *en route* to an evening engagement. And having time to cut the grass when the weather was right, rather than because it was my day off and if I didn't do it today I would have to wait a week for the next opportunity!

Inevitably invitations began to arrive. The prospect of adding a newly retired cleric to one's list of visiting preachers was a great temptation for some clergy and even more so for churchwardens facing an interregnum. So at an early stage I decided that the only way to protect myself and my new-found freedom was to strike off whole stretches of the diary when I was 'off', and concentrate my acceptance of invitations into those weeks and months when I was 'on'. This ensures periods of freedom to holiday or entertain, or to play the grandparent.

We are not, however, floating worshippers. We soon settled into a church, where we find spiritual nourishment and warmth on the occasions when we are not on the road or preaching elsewhere. We may not be in our pews every Sunday, but the church fellowship know we are supporting them and ready to help out if needed. And it is lovely to have a parish to which to belong and a ministry for which to pray. We owe the church a great deal, and, what is more, they allow us to sit together in the congregation as husband and wife, a new pleasure after all these years of being seated at different ends of the church on a Sunday.

We can also entertain, not lavishly or in parties, but we now have time to invite someone to drop in for a meal, or if they call unexpectedly we can down tools and give

ourselves to welcoming them in without wondering how
we can get rid of them before the next engagement is due.
And I think they in their turn are rather pleased to meet
the relaxed hospitality that goes with all the time in the
world.

This is particularly true of the family who over the years
have become used to finding that whenever they came to
see us they were competing with busy diaries and a round
of interviews and outside engagements. It used to make us
feel very guilty and inadequate as parents, but now that is
all a thing of the past. Now we have to fit in with their
busy schedules!

We also have more time to pray, as distinct from being
at services. We have always tried jealously to guard our
morning times of prayer, but this has only been possible
by dint of disciplined use of alarm clocks. Now we can
overrun with a clear conscience, in the knowledge that
no secretaries or telephone calls will be making their
demands on our time the moment the clock strikes nine,
or even earlier. Our partnership does not of course end
there. Because we have the whole day to share, we can plan
the household tasks between us; go to the supermarket
together, hang out the washing, do the garden together,
divide up some of the chores, so that they are not all left
to my wife.

I am often asked if I miss my old job, and the answer is
certainly yes. I miss the action, the information, the adren-
alin situations . . . the gossip! No, not in any bad way, but
the vast flow of news about people and parishes, the
births, marriages and deaths, the welfare of those who
have been ill, and all that has gone into the contents of our
praying over so many years. We do hear a good deal of
news, but not nearly so promptly, and that is something we
have had to learn to let go of. We retain contact through
many letters and cards, and that is some compensation,
but the fact is that we are no longer on the job and we
cannot be entitled to know everything that is going on,

least of all on General Synod committees and suchlike. So our prayers and concerns have become much more localized, including neighbours and their needs as well as parishioners and clergy.

When first we contemplated the prospect of retirement, one of the things my wife said to me was that I would now be able to prepare some new sermons! It was not meant unkindly, just a comment on the luxury of having time to do a better job. This too has been a rewarding opportunity. The three-hour service on Good Friday was a case in point. Instead of working over so much familiar ground, I was able to start over again with a completely new theme and give whole days to preparation. The result was that I was fired as never before with the excitement of finding out truths from the Scriptures that were new to me, and the service took on a special significance for me. Whether it did for the congregation I could not say, but I hope it did. No one could complain that they had heard it all before!

So here we are in our first year of a new life, what I prefer to call our penultimate spell of Christian ministry. Our final spell will be in heaven. We have no idea how long we shall be allowed to stay here or how long we shall be together in our Christian discipleship. All I can say is that it is as blissful as it has been cracked up to be and we enjoy every minute of it. And our love for one another and of our Lord seems to grow as the days go by. I hope I am not being too starry-eyed, but that's how it is at the moment. Thanks be to God.

## Linda Taylor

I had always warned my husband that I would be ready to 'draw stumps' when I had turned sixty-five, and mercifully he took me at my word. It is exactly forty years since we were married in St Paul's, Cambridge, and here we are back again! And on reflection I know that I was beginning to experience some limitations. There was a continual

tiredness, sight and hearing problems making themselves
felt when one least wanted them, twinges and aches which
made things an effort, memory letting one down, blood
pressure problems, an irregular heartbeat, and the realization that routine chores were taking longer and would
leave one more tired than usual. I might still be capable of
having a good idea but I lacked the energy to put it into
action! I had always known that my stamina was entirely
dependent on the Lord and on other people's prayers, but
now I felt I was becoming a positive liability!

Speaking as a wife, I would estimate that I spent the best
part of a year preparing for retirement: gradually pulling
out of committees and responsibilities in my husband's
diocese and, at the same time, compiling lists and information for our successors; I went on a term's computer
course at the local college and tried to think ahead what
we would need, getting records onto floppy disk; sifting
through every file and folder of fifteen years' work and
further back, in our personal files. I knew about the
problems in sorting out paperwork and possessions for
deceased parents, and did not want to leave that sort of
legacy to our family. I remember filling over four black
plastic sacks with the shreddings of accumulated junk! But
it paid off to update the admin. – preparing the address
labels for Christmas; the 'LISTORG' database for sending
our change of address to each organization, bank, medical,
legal or ecclesiastical group, journal and charity; working
out how to survive on a pension with no 'expenses cov-
ered'; what we needed and what we could do without.

Then to adapt and plan for a move from an eighteen-
roomed house to a nine-roomed vicarage style house
again. I was mentally humping furniture about for weeks,
and sloughing off onto family and charity anything 'not
wanted on voyage'. Then there was the need to plan for a
trouble-free household (is there such a thing?) and an easily
maintained garden where we could enjoy our love of bird-
watching, and invite our many friends to come and relax.

Our Ruby Wedding suggestion was to invite generous inquirers to give us those 'priceless rubies' which are inch-square pieces of sticky paper with our Queen's head on them ... first-class stamps! ... since the invitations and demands which my husband receives almost daily come without a stamped, addressed envelope. Retirement is an expensive business!

---

### Moving Day

Like sloughing off a skin
In which I have grown for years,
I leave this house.

Stripped of my personal marks,
It echoes with memories
Of joys and sorrows,
And waits with open heart
To greet its new inhabitants.

And I, temporarily
Possessing nothing, wait
To grow into another home,
Prepare for fresh encounter
With the Holy One.

Written by Ann Lewin on 1 March 1996, after the removal van had left, and as she waited for a phone call to say she could pick up the keys to her new retirement home.

## CLARE CLUCAS

For me the secret of finding a new identity in retirement has been to learn to practise acceptance. I have had to realize that the years have passed and that I must change. For one thing, my husband and I moved to a much smaller home in a different town, partly because the congregational church we had attended closed down. We had to learn to cope with increasing physical limitations and discover a new lifestyle. Part of this new way of life has been learning to accept help when it is needed and being prepared to adapt.

The transition to retirement was a smooth one for me. In my earlier years raising my three children was my priority, but then as they grew independent I took on some paid work at my husband's office. Although I retired at sixty I went back into the office for several periods of a few months to help out when an employee was on sick leave. I enjoyed the routine of work, but I missed, and continue to miss my children, who now live away.

When my husband retired several years after me, I felt I lost my freedom to a degree and had to adjust to a new situation. Over the years his health has deteriorated, leaving him with partial sight, deafness and heart and kidney problems. So part of my role in retirement has been to care for him and cultivate patience in myself.

One aspect of retirement I have found to be greatly rewarding has been my training and work in a caring organization. I had always done voluntary work in the town where we lived before retiring, but this was a new interest. The on-going training we receive is very stimulating. I also help with the church guild, which is mainly attended by elderly women. This, too, entails much pastoral work.

### COLONEL HARDY, SA, AGED SEVENTY-FIVE

The Salvationists' religion incorporates much that conflicts with the normal experiences of old age, mental and physical. It advocates a strident sunniness, positive action and a dramatic interpretation of, and obedience to, orders. The orders either filter down from the Army's own High Command or are given directly to a soldier by God himself, and a lot of the excitement of life devolves from the receipt and operation of these instructions. But life – even the most kindly understood life – being what it is, the year arrives when the orders officially cease and, since one has never smoked, drunk, or had much money, or liberty to worry about one's own affairs, and is thus likely to be exceptionally healthy at seventy, one has a problem.

The traditional virtue of elderly Christians, *benig-nitas*, a sort of exuding of long-amassed prayer, is more likely to be the reward of the religious introvert than the average Salvationist during the interim between his being relieved of his command and his being 'promoted to glory', as the obituaries in the *War Cry* put it. For the average Salvationist is a person of stir and movement, a spiritual *possibliste* for whom inaction is unnatural and uncaring. Of course, like all religious organisations, the Salvation Army says that there is no real retirement from its ranks and that members soldier-on until the end. Yet when the day comes when '(R)' has to be placed after one's name in the List, no amount of lip-service to careers which only death can halt is able to conceal the fact that it produces a shock in many a life geared to action and selfless involvement.

> A contribution from Ronald Blythe's *The View in Winter: Reflections on Old Age* (Penguin Books 1981).

## THE REVD MICHAEL AND DOROTHY HOY

For us retirement has only just become a reality. Having served in the Anglican ministry, with the sustenance of God's grace and the gift of good health, the idea of *early* retirement had not entered the equation of life. Retirement was something that would happen at the age of sixty-five: out there in the future. There must come a time, however, when the future begins to make itself heard and demand attention. In our case this happened with the invitation to a pre-retirement conference in 1993. Initially this seemed to be a premature event, but once we were immersed in it we realized it was not too soon to begin thinking about the practical and psychological implications of retirement. Maybe the psychology could wait, but the practicalities could not, because we had soon to seek a place to which to retire. This involved finding the first home of our own, since we had always been in 'tied' accommodation. We recalled the advice of a former Bishop of Ripon: 'When you have one foot in the grave, you should have the other one at a bus stop'!

So we moved into a phase when praying and looking for the right location became a new occupation – exciting and demanding. In retrospect it was the right timing for us to begin the search for a location two years before retirement. It was also right to begin 'sorting' our belongings more than twelve months before retirement. Even then we ended up with more pressure than was desirable in the final stages of packing. A major consideration for us was contraction: four bedrooms, a study, a separate dining room, a pantry and a 'store' room had to give way to two and a half bedrooms, no study, no pantry, no store and just a dining 'area'. You cannot put a quart into a pint pot! Peering round piles of boxes, we have not yet discovered whether the contraction has been sufficiently ruthless.

It is really too early to write about the psychological and spiritual adjustments which retirement will involve. A time of taking stock and rediscovery and re-alignment lies ahead of us. There are old interests to develop and there is the excitement of exploring new ones. In terms of ministry we have an open mind, knowing only that the Lord surely has his mind on work for us to do. We shall put up our antennae and see what signals we get!

It has been a welcome thing for both of us to experience the end of life lived under the pressure of constraints – of deadlines, appointments and demanding situations – and to have the freedom to choose how we use our time and energy. At the same time we have lost a life in which we had ready-made relationships and a spiritual 'home' provided for us. Now we shall need to seek out new friends and look for a congregation where we shall take our place, more in the pew than in the pulpit.

## REG WYATT

The transition to retirement three years ago was for me smooth and without stress or regret. This was partly because my career job, although satisfying, was not my only interest and it did not dominate my life; it was partly also because I was encouraged to attend a pre-retirement course, which provided helpful guidelines. Thus it was a genuine transition, which I viewed as a change of role, not as a sad end to a fulfilling career. Furthermore, I was fully aware that retirement would allow me to pursue interests for which I had previously had little time. So there was no concern over how I would fill my days; my problem now is rather that there does not seem to be enough time.

The opportunities I have had to continue my professional work on a casual basis, pursuing geological research from time to time and writing papers for publication, has been a helpful factor. I have also had opportunities to do other things – I am now secretary to the church PCC and to a local Christian trust. I am able to spend much more time tending the garden with my wife. I continue as a volunteer on the Great Central Steam Railway. Shopping and domestic duties, though not the most enjoyable of activities, are part of my schedule. And I walk when I can. I enjoy being active and having constructive things to do.

# 2

# Finding New Priorities

There tends to be a strong element of ambivalence mixed in with people's feelings about being older. We make a virtue out of 'not feeling our age' and 'looking ten years younger'. Many people seem preoccupied with maintaining a youthful appearance, which is hardly surprising in a society which appears to celebrate youth and has spawned a vast industry dedicated to the task of keeping wrinkles and grey hair at bay.

Old age is portrayed as a barren, inhospitable country to which no one would choose to travel. Is it any wonder, then, that we take a circuitous route on the journey towards our final years, selecting various detours of denial until we plainly can no longer ignore the truth that we have arrived at old age? Yet there is great damage done in our refusal to embrace willingly our own ageing. We miss out on the genuine benefits which a perspective from later life can offer. Of course it is true to say that we retain the essence of our selves – our personalities, our identities which have been shaped throughout the life-course – but retirement does bring a fresh dimension, an altered focus.

The academic study of ageing, gerontology, has invested considerable energy in researching the new values and ambitions people adopt and develop through retirement. Once the tasks of earlier adult life have been accomplished (careers have been established, families raised), the older person need no longer be preoccupied with the need to build for the future. Thus freed from these demands, retired people have the time and space to give deeper thought to the meaning of life. They also have the benefit of amassed experience of the world to help shed light on their search for truth.

Many older people, looking back on the things which absorbed their youthful energies and passions, can often find themselves wondering why they considered these things to be of such significance. The things which now seem to matter most in life can be very different. Older people seem to become less bothered about their image and the way in which those around them view them. They no longer wish to hide aspects of their personalities which might be considered less acceptable. Older men, for instance, often develop a greater awareness of their feelings and express a previously unseen softness and tenderness in their relationships. Another characteristic that can appear in later life is a greater tolerance and understanding of people and actions that might previously have been condemned. Older people have learned that life is rarely black and white and they often show tremendous skills of empathy. Faith has deepened and matured and shines from them in ways which give encouragement to those they meet.

The way in which an individual handles their later years depends a great deal, of course, on how they have spent their earlier lives. Contentment lies in store for those who feel reasonably satisfied with all that they have achieved. Those who look back and remember only failure and disappointment, on the other hand, can become absorbed in feelings of guilt and depression; these are the people who find it difficult in retirement to look outwards towards the needs of others.

The older people featured in this chapter vary in age and background, and this is reflected in their comments on retirement. Through their stories we can see the process whereby later life calls us to reassess our priorities and shift focus.

### HENRI NOUWEN AND WALTER GAFFNEY

Perhaps it is detachment, a gentle 'letting-go', that allows the elderly to break through the illusions of immortality and smile at all the urgencies and emergencies of their past life. When everything is put in its proper place, there is time to greet the true reasons for living.

Hope and humor can give rise to a new vision. Once in a while we meet an old man or woman looking far beyond the boundaries of their human existence into a light that seems to embrace him or her with gentleness and kindness. Once in a while we hear about this light as about a friendly host calling us home . . . .

The vision which grows in aging can lead us beyond the limitations of our human self. It is a vision that makes us not only detach ourselves from preoccupation with the past but also from the importance of the present. It is a vision which invites us to a total, fearless surrender in which the distinction between life and death slowly loses its pain.

Quoted from *Aging: The Fulfillment of Life*, by Henri J. M. Nouwen and Walter J. Gaffney (Doubleday 1976).

### AMY BASNETT

I never thought about being older. I would say it just comes to you. I certainly never dreaded retiring from work because I have always kept myself busy.

I was a baker. My sister and I were both confectioners and had a shop. I went to classes to learn my trade, though our parents were in the business too. I met Joe, my husband, through amateur dramatics. I married at nineteen, when Joe was twenty-one. Not long afterwards he joined the forces, despite efforts by his boss (he worked for a newspaper as a linotype operator) to have him exempted. Joe was away in the Far East during the war. He left in 1942, when our son Harry was only sixteen months. We were a one-parent family really. Joe did not smoke, so when he received his cigarette ration he would exchange it for sweets to send home – mind you, they never tasted good! I coped well during the war because I was involved with everything that went on at church.

Church has always been my life. My father was Sunday School Superintendent and was given a medal for twenty-five years' service. As children, we always went to church in the morning, Sunday School in the afternoon and church again in the evening. Back then we paid pew rents! Church was more of a family thing. My son sang in the choir and my husband was churchwarden. My sister and I started the tradition of the Rose Queen at the church, back in 1957. We felt it would be something for the children – the Queen and her retinue appear on seven occasions at important services through the year. I have organized it ever since, though this is my last year and no one has been found to take over from me.

When Joe returned from the war I worked as a confectioner three days a week. Joe and his brother set up a wholesale greengrocery business together. It took Harry a long time to take to Joe. I would tell Harry to ask his father's permission for things, but he would not talk to him. Joe died suddenly in 1968 at the age of fifty-two. I was only forty-nine so I have been a widow now for many years. For the last fifteen years of my working life I was a school cook. I worked at an 'open air' school for sickly children. When I had been there a while it became a school for maladjusted youngsters, mainly from children's homes. They would try to be cheeky with me, but I wouldn't let them have their dinner until they said 'please' and 'thank you'!

My priorities have changed since retiring. My family are

a top priority. My son and his children and grandchildren all live a few miles away. I see them all regularly. Each Wednesday I collect my great-grandson and great grand-daughter from school and nursery and take them for tea at Harry's house. I have my great-grandchildren to stay at my home and I enjoy their company. But my relatives know that I would never allow them to come before my church commitments. And if I couldn't look after myself any longer, I would not choose to live with them. I love them, but I don't want to live in their pockets; I would rather have my own life! I serve on several committees – Christian Aid, Churches Together, and the Children's Society (from which I received a long-service certificate).

I have lived in Darwen all my life, so I know many of the local people – too many, I sometimes think! I would never want to leave the town. I live in the centre which means friends can call on me when they are passing. I moved to this house in 1939 because it was next door to Joe's parents, and I have lived here ever since. Daytimes are your own when you are retired, but I am out most evenings. If ever I have a night in, I think 'thank good-ness'! I also have holidays on my own. Being widowed so young, I have had plenty of time to get used to my own company.

It is sad to see how much Darwen has declined over the years, since the cotton mills began to close in the 1950s. They employed so many local people. We also had two pits locally which shut down.

Being busy has helped make my retirement happy. I enjoy good health and have always been a positive, outgoing person. I don't feel retirement has changed me – old age will hit me some day! I am seventy-seven now. A lot of people are afraid of losing their homes, but you don't know what you might have to face up to.

Looking back on my life, I don't think I would do any-thing differently. I don't have anything on my conscience. I could never have lived with broken relationships.

## ELISABETH CHURCH

The exciting journey of faith does not stand still. We cannot be boxed in by a decision taken long ago. We see that there are many paths to God. People find Him in all sorts of ways, and they come to faith by many routes, often by a slow dawning of light, sometimes by a sudden Damascus Road experience, as long as they find Him, all is valid. To have a closed mind means to perish.

For me, in old age, the world is opening up more and more. I am aware of the dignity and value of the whole human race. I glimpse the wonder of creation from the vast incomprehensible galaxies and stars to the tiniest flower and insect, the raindrop on a leaf or the unbelievable beauty of a spider's web woven in the frost.

As a young Christian for many years I felt I could only worship in a certain sort of church and a certain sort of community. They had to be 'like-minded' and 'my sort', even my social background.

In my middle years I used to love a hearty service with little pause for silence – I just joined in regardless. Gradually the need to worship grew – if possible without wandering thoughts pressing in on me, and now I really try to pray the prayers and mean the words of the hymns. We hear people criticising the clergy and many hunt around trying to find the perfect church. There is no perfect church and clergy are human. It seems to me that the need is to attend and to think more about what you can contribute to the act of worship rather than what you can get out of it . . . .

Regarding issues of morality, liberal ideas are flooding in and much that I hold dear is being swept away. Chastity is one of these. I find in myself a certain hardness and judgemental attitude which can take over, possibly because it hurts so deeply to see the decline in moral standards in our country today. For myself I feel I must keep the standards which I feel are right but not condemn or judge or turn aside from those whose values differ from mine . . . .

In youth I was dogmatic, dismissive of other people's views and at times insensitive. I pray now for a growing sensitivity and above all love for all mankind.

From *For Ever Jubilant: The Adventure of Ageing* by
Elisabeth Church (1993).

## THE REVD NICK CARR

I became a Christian over fifty-five years ago and, after six years in the armed forces, and on completing my university course at Cambridge, I worked for sixteen years in the family's biscuit firm, Carrs of Carlisle. Following the shattering experience of being made redundant, due to a takeover, I went to theological college and was duly ordained in the Anglican Church. After four years as a curate the call came to join the Overseas Missionary Fellowship as Home Director. I served in this capacity for six years and then was appointed Minister at Large, which led to a very wide preaching ministry for a further eight years. For some years I was privileged to be a regular speaker at the Keswick Convention and served as a council member and trustee for thirty years. On retiring, I became editor, for eight years, of a Christian magazine called *The Overcomer*.

Joy and I have now been married for forty-six years, and have four boys and three girls, all of whom are now married. Between them they have presented us with twenty-three grandchildren. We have been tremendously blessed, as all of our seven children have put their trust in the Lord Jesus.

As I look back over the years, I am very conscious of the truly wonderful way in which the Lord has led me. The older I grow, the more I have to look back at his grace, and the greater confidence it gives me in regards to the future. Every phase of my life has been a preparation for the next phase, so I am sure that the coming years will be the final preparation for the fullness of the life still to come.

So what of the future? I have now been retired for over ten years and gradually my ministry is being changed. I have just retired from very close links with the Keswick Convention and the time has come to pass on the editorship of *The Overcomer* to my successor. I still have many preaching engagements and run a weekly Bible study group, but there is now more time for other activities. I will be able to see more of the family. Already there is more time to pray. I hope to write more letters to missionaries and from time to time write articles. There will also be more time for Bible study and reading. It will be good to watch more cricket in the summer and more rugby football in the winter! In fact the future looks very exciting.

Three years ago, Joy and I were involved in a very serious accident. We drove right under a huge tanker at a speed of about sixty-four mph on a motorway. The roof of the car was shaved right off just above our heads, but apart from some bruising we were both unscathed. This was truly a miracle and certainly our guardian angels had been working overtime that night. What effect did this have on me? When I saw the wreck of the car next morning, after a night in hospital for observation, I realized that if I had not woken up in the ambulance, I would have woken up in the nearer presence of my Lord. I realized in a far deeper way that there was no fear of death to those who have come to faith in him. There may be a fear of dying, as we have been given the instinct of self-preservation, but we have his promises: 'My grace is sufficient for you' and 'I will never leave you nor forsake you'.

There has been another important reaction. I have come to realize that the next meeting at which I am asked to preach is the most important one. It might be my last! I may be wrong but I believe that it has brought about a greater cutting edge to my ministry. I now find increasingly the importance of living one day at a time. There is a daily need for repentance; a daily need to be filled afresh with the Holy Spirit and a daily commitment to his service.

In my 'quiet time' this morning I came across this passage:

> Be dressed ready for service and keep your lamps burning, like men waiting for their master to return from a wedding banquet, so that when he comes and knocks they can immediately open the door for him. It will be good for those servants whose master finds them watching when he comes. (Luke 12.35–7)

I do not know what is going to happen in my life before God either takes me home or comes to catch me up to be with him for ever. I can only live one day at a time and it is no use worrying about the future. To quote Hudson Taylor, 'Satan would have us try today to bear tomorrow's burden with only today's grace'. My responsibility is to pray that whatever he allows to take place in my life, I may act and respond in such a way that it will bring honour and glory to his name. The final answer is clear:

> he will 'transform our lowly bodies so that they will be like his glorious body' (Philippians 3.21) and 'We shall see him as he is' (1 John 3.3). Surely I must rest daily on this glorious and certain hope.

## REG WYATT

My first priority, both before and after retirement, has been to love, worship and serve the Lord to the best of my ability. The extent to which I have succeeded has, I confess, varied from time to time. This point of focus, nevertheless, has not changed.

In terms of attitudes and outlook, my change of focus from earlier adulthood was more to do with becoming a Christian (at the age of thirty-five) than anything else. The 'new man' has new priorities. Thus, subsequent events, including retirement and growth in 'worldly wisdom', have had less impact. As a Christian, I feel very uneasy about the world and its values, most of which are quite contrary to those of the believer. Were it not for my faith, I would be very cynical about the ways of the world! Certainly, however, worldly wisdom and life experience have enabled me to become more realistic about our society and less dogmatic in my views. I think I am more tolerant and understanding of others, realizing that bizarre behaviour may stem from traumatic experiences. I am more ready to be a mediator and a peacemaker. I now see that there is a time to remain silent. I am much less disposed to be strait-jacketed by other people's expectations of me. I have a better judgement of my own worth. What a difference from the introverted, self-conscious, self-deprecating, self-centred, anxious young man I was in my twenties!

## MARY THOMAS

The transition from paid employment to organizing one's own life should be taken very seriously. When older adolescents talk about gaining freedom they mean getting away from teachers, parents and indeed anyone with authority over them. When older people envisage freedom they imagine escaping from humdrum working lives. They seldom give constructive thought to the future.

For professional people the freedom of retirement brings the opportunity to spend their handsome pensions on things for which they have had little time. In our class society, made up of 'them and us', however, 'they' have never really tasted freedom and a large majority will never experience it.

Being a Christian, I possible see things differently. Older age offers freedom from important responsibilities. Whatever one's status, whether widowed, or the parent of children with their own families, or single, the positive goal in life has largely gone. From birth up until this stage in life we have been responsible for and answerable to at least one other person. This can mean that, though most older people visit the doctor for a very good reason, many a condition is exacerbated by loneliness and boredom.

During my working life as a teacher, I spent much time in very deprived areas. I remember well the way in which parents in such places were treated by society, by authority. And I think that the less well educated older person is treated in similar ways. After a lifetime of never sticking up for themselves, what hope have they now in their more vulnerable time of life?

Eight years ago, I founded the Dark Horse Venture in Liverpool. I felt that many older people in the city were both bored and lonely. Our aim is to help them set goals for themselves. Through embarking on new activities – whether learning a skill, starting an exercise programme or taking up voluntary work – they find new confidence and motivation. Many make new friends and broaden their social circle. I have seen so much positive change in that an increasing number of people are now recognizing that spending time in an interesting, enjoyable occupation is the solution to the problems of many retired people. General practitioners are referring their older patients to leisure centres for supervised personal programmes and residential homes are providing activities other than Bingo. It is happening slowly, but it is happening.

The message of the Dark Horse Venture is spreading. Our ideas have been taken up throughout the UK, Northern and Southern Ireland, in Australia, New Zealand, Canada, Zimbabwe, South Africa, Liberia, Spain, Portugal, Luxembourg, Denmark, Sweden and Hungary. In each country the problems of older age are similar.

Having myself reached the stage of 'older age', there are several points which really worry me:

- Why can't people realize that the main difference between older people and younger people is simply that the older people have lived longer than the younger?

- Why do people not realize that anyone who lives long enough will one day be old?

- Why do we abuse so many older people by discussing who we should, or should not, care for in old age?

- If young people complain about their taxes being spent on older people, will they feel the same when it comes to caring for older members of their own families, or indeed when they themselves grow old?

Many of the people now over sixty were brought up in a strict Christian environment. They were taught to understand the difference between right and wrong, to know the meaning of respect and to show care for others. Now these things seem largely gone and their absence is mourned.

The opportunity for learning, sharing, thinking and praying should surely be provided as of right in every city, town, village and hamlet, and for each retired person. Only then will people come to realize what life is all about and that God loves every man, woman and child, unconditionally. Only then will we see that life is to be enjoyed and lived to the full, to the end.

## CARMEN SMITH

### Magnificat Moments

After fifty years of religious life, I have returned to live in the novitiate (which I've learned to call 'the house of initial formation'). It has been a time of happy renewal – a second 'first' years of commitment and community. All the freshness and enthusiasm of first beginning in the Society has touched the steadiness and comfortable ease of a life lived and given, lived and given during these fifty years. In quiet celebration of our vocation – knowing again that God chose first – I have delighted to watch the initial formation of today's young women and to share their prayer. Through contact with their sensitivity for the suffering of the poor, I have become more aware of the real meaning of concern for the marginalised – the lonely, the sick, the abused, the hungry.

Somehow living with these younger women has made me more able to grow into old age without fear, without regrets, without resistance. I'd thought that when I was older it would be a time to pass on to the young what I've known and loved in the Society. In many ways I've found the young pass on to me their vision of the world and its need, their hope for the future and their dreams of how hope and faith can acquire a 'local habitation and a name'. So our treasures become not hand-me-downs, but hand-me-ups . . . .

In these later years, there is a time for the steady response of *magnificat* to all that life has brought of joy and pain, darkness and light, springtime and winter of the spirit. This is the time to quietly, gently absorb the mystery of life and to capture wonder.

From *On the Way Home: Reflections for Old Age*, ed. Frances Makower and Joan Faber (Darton, Longman and Todd 1994).

## 3

# Assessing and Learning from the Past

One aspect of being older which younger people often find frustrating is the tendency among many retired people to dwell on the past. It can appear that some have lost the ability to live in the present or to look to the future, so obsessed are they with looking back over their previous lives. They express a cloying nostalgia over a bygone era and fail to acknowledge the improvements that have come about over the years.

There are tremendous benefits in spending time looking back over our lives and taking stock. In fact, it is something we do from time to time whatever our age. Writing in the journal *The Way* in April 1996, Eugene Bianchi says that the reminiscences of older people form part of the great tradition within Christianity of 'story-telling' as a means of building faith. Story-telling can help heal memories which could otherwise lead to bitterness. It can also help older people recognize skills and achievements from their past which might help in the future. Harvesting memories can help cultivate inner resources. This story-telling can shed light on the meaning of a person's life, benefiting younger listeners as well as adding to their own understanding. The testimony of the contributors to this chapter bears witness to God's faithfulness and guidance over a life span lasting up to a century.

The use we make of our reflections can vary, though. We can accept uncritically the unravelling of our destinies or we can look back on them with an eye to drawing from them lessons to help us cope with the situations we now face. Contributors to this book have often used what they have learned of God's kindness and trustworthiness in the past to help them face current challenges.

Implicit in this understanding of the role of reminiscence is the assumption that there will be listeners. Part of the intrinsic value of being able to relate your story is the sense that you are conveying information and insights to another, younger person, to whom they may be of genuine benefit. The presence of an audience transforms the sterility of nostalgia into the dynamism of wisdom. Churches provide a good context in which the generations can learn from one another, where younger people can help their seniors to make sense of their memories, while taking from their conversations with them lessons for their own lives.

The long and the short of it is that it helps to have people with whom to share recollections of the past. Those whose memories contain much which may give rise to sadness and regret need loving support. Those for whom looking back is a happier process require friends with whom to rejoice. Story-telling is a central part of our walk of faith. And as contributors to this book so rightly say, the blessing for the children of God is that the past can be left securely in his hands. For failures we can find forgiveness. For uncertainty he can give peace. There is no need for morose preoccupation with the sins of yesteryear. With God each day is a fresh beginning and an opportunity for growth.

## DOROTHY SHERRY

Like most old people I tend to look back at my life, and I rejoice over the many and varied areas of Christian work to which God called me. I soon learned that 'the place of God's appointment was the only place of blessing'.

I was twenty-six years of age when my father remarried and I was free to begin life! God led me into the ranks of the Church Army and I spent three happy years doing mission work in East and Mid-Suffolk. My next 'call' sent me to Northern Nigeria to work with leper children and motherless babies. I was also involved with village evangelism. Twelve years later I was back in England and waiting for God to guide me.

In 1954 I went to a home for the elderly as assistant matron and in 1955 took charge of a home for fifteen residents in Bacup, Lancashire. I stayed there for eighteen happy years until I retired in 1973.

Retirement did not change my life very much. I had elderly friends and neighbours who needed love and care. I spent much of my time looking after them. I have just celebrated my eighty-seventh birthday. I do not feel old or think or act old. I am blessed with a good memory. I live alone, yet I am never alone. When I feel afraid I go upstairs and read a card, given to me in 1973, which has the words: 'I will never abandon you, I will never leave you'. That gives me the reassurance I need.

I feel age has made me more tolerant. I can even listen to friends who repeat the same story over and over! I find that strangers take my arm and help me across the road. They open heavy doors for me when I am out shopping. I do not mind being awake at four o'clock in the morning. I make a cup of tea and settle down to Bible reading and quiet time.

St Paul wrote: 'Nothing can separate us from the love of God'. Yes, God loves me, he supplies all my needs and as the hymn says, 'Your glory and might are beyond us to tell, and yet in the heart of the humble you dwell'.

## PALMIRA DE OROVIO

Treasure

Archaeologists attach great importance to the discovery of antiquities. Reflecting on this and on the current interest in television programmes like *The Antiques Roadshow*, it has occurred to me that we – the elderly – can discover similar treasures in our own lives. Life has been a great adventure . . . things that seemed of little worth have been shown to have great value, just as uranium, once considered a waste product, has been found to be a source of atomic energy.

Coming to terms with ourselves on the eve of our dissolution, we discover with pride the riches we have accumulated throughout our lives. Working, like the best tapestry-makers, from behind – a stitch here, a knot there, using the colours God has given us – and when we turn it over

. . . a miracle! One day we shall see the result and will marvel at what God has done in us and through us.

We must never lose heart; our latent energy is greater than we realise: having suffered we have learned patience; knowing our weakness, we can think more kindly of others; being used to discomfort, we can handle inconvenience. The wonder of each new day makes us optimistic and we expect the best: someone will smile at us, or repeat what we have not been able to hear; someone will give a helping hand on the stairs, or say something kind.

We delight in it all on awakening, thank God and try to do the same for others. At the end of the day, let us not ask whether we have been made happy, but rather, what have we done to make others happy today?

From *On the Way Home: Reflections for Old Age*, ed. Frances Makower and Joan Faber (Darton, Longman and Todd 1994).

## THE REVD PAT AND MARION ASHE

One of the things we learned from our many moves within the ordained Anglican ministry (six in twenty-five years) was not to hang on to the past. When we left a parish, it was 'hands off'. Any links we kept were on the basis of friendship and not our former role within the church.

I was privileged to have Cuthbert Bardsley (later Bishop of Coventry) as my first rector at Woolwich, and then at St Mark's Kennington I learnt much from the vicar, the Revd Wallace Bird, lessons which I began to put into practice in Blindley Heath. Otley was perhaps the biggest challenge. What I inherited from my Yorkshire grand-mother, a Routh from near Beverley, helped me to overcome my Southern accent, and once we 'broke through', the years there were very happy.

Leamington Spa saw the beginning of the work of Project Vietnam Orphans. It began at a meeting of eight men. The vast number of orphaned and abandoned children in the world did not deter us – 'Let's not be put off by the millions,' we agreed, 'let's try and rescue one.' The organization was born. We got over a hundred children adopted into Christian homes, and it is lovely to meet some of them, now in their twenties. Perhaps some of the ones we could not bring out will remember those young women with fair hair and blue eyes, PVO's nurses, who crossed half the world to pick them up when they cried, to wipe their noses, to show them love, because they had the Spirit of Jesus in their hearts.

At Church Stretton, with three churches to look after, we found it impossible to cope with both the parish and the work of PVO – the adoptions in this country, recruitment of nurses, correspondence, and occasional visits to Vietnam. We took the rather frightening step of faith and moved from the security of a parish with a seven-bedroomed rectory, into a tiny bungalow (there were nine of us) in Godalming, with no regular income. Marion did night duty in a hospital and God wonderfully provided for our needs.

Probably the most important answers to prayer in our experience have been when we were totally helpless. To give an example, when we finally had to leave Vietnam before the Vietcong took over, we were faced by an apparently insoluble problem. We had a message from the British Ambassador that we should leave the country. But we had sixteen babies waiting for their release papers. We could not take them with us – we could not stay – we had no one with whom to leave them. We could see no way out. Our reading that night was from the book of Exodus, about the children of Israel leaving Egypt. They had a similarly intractable problem – the Red Sea in front and the Egyptian army behind. God spoke to Moses (Exodus 14.13): 'Stand still and see the salvation of the Lord'.

The next morning the war correspondent from the *Daily Mail* knocked on our gate. He said, 'We have a plane coming in the day after tomorrow to take you and the children out.' I said, 'We have sixteen babies.' 'The plane will hold 150, so see what you can do!' Then there was a series of 'after-miracles', and 101 children came out on the plane.

The work continued in Thailand, and we formed Christian Outreach. Another 'hand-over' took place when we retired and Roy Clarke took over the chairmanship. We let go and only offered advice when asked. It has been a real joy to see the work expanding in Cambodia, Sudan, Eritrea, Mozambique, Ruanda, and now once more back in Vietnam.

So, what about retirement? At first we felt guilty for not knowing who lived in every house around us! But we soon found there was much to be done. I became Honorary Chaplain to Losely Place and the Estate St Francis Littleton, the Estate Church, and to the staff at Guildway. I also assist with the Christian Cancer Help Centre which meets twice a month at Loseley. Most Sundays I am asked to help in various churches in the area. It is a rare event to find a day with nothing in the diary.

Now our days are getting numbered – Marion is seventy-five and I am eighty-one. We are facing the fact that physically we are not immortal – one of us is going to be left. The house is getting too much for Marion, and the garden too big for me. So we keep asking for 'guidance'. Should we sell the house and move to a smaller one, or a flat? Can we face the upheaval of moving? We have no clear answer yet. Our main resource is not where we live but our certainty that God loves us. We look back with enormous gratitude for the way he has led us through the years, and for all the love that has surrounded us from our family and friends. So we want to keep close to him – Jesus, 'dear name, the rock on which I build, my shield and hiding place, my never failing treasury filled with boundless stores of grace'.

It is futile to try and imagine what the next life will be like. We shall be entering into a different element. The grub at the bottom of the pond in mud and water could never imagine what it is like to become a dragonfly in a different element of air. But we know that underneath are the everlasting arms (Deuteronomy 33.27) and that nothing can separate us from the love of God (Romans 8.39).

—————

Lord, my Father,
when I look back over my life,
I am ashamed to remember
how many times I failed you
when I was presented with opportunities for service.

I recall the excuses:
it was not convenient;
it might prove too costly in time and effort;
I had other things to do;
I was not feeling well;
there were other things more important;
and so on, and so on.

I recall with shame
that many of the opportunities
did not call for any great sacrifice.
You did not ask for anything
I could not do.

Sometimes I looked
for the big, the spectacular thing to do
and I missed what I considered beneath me
when it was what you wanted
and I could have done it.
I should have had more faith in you,
more love for my neighbour.

Dear Lord,
show me how I can still serve you,
even through the limitations of my age
and energy.

From A *Pensioner's Prayer Book* by J. H. Speed
(John Paul the Preacher's Press 1981).


## HAROLD SMITH

I was a hundred in January 1996. In the Christian nursing home where I live with my wife, Doris, we had a party. My son took the telegram the Queen sent me to be framed. People ask me the secret of living long. I feel I have lived to this great age because throughout my life I have relied on prayer and remembered to 'keep the Sabbath day holy'.

I first started to pray when I was a young child at school. I always struggled with my arithmetic. Then, one day, a lady came to speak to us about prayer. She told us that prayer was not just for adults, that if we had problems we children should bring them to the Lord and ask for his help. I prayed each day about my arithmetic. I well remember the time when I was leaving school, at the age of fourteen. The headmaster asked to see me. 'Smith,' he said, 'a miracle has happened. You were bottom of the class in arithmetic and now you are top!'

Ever since then prayer has mattered a lot to me. Now I am no longer able to go to church I still pray, here in my room. In fact, if anything, prayer is more important to me than ever. And now Doris can no longer pray, I pray for her.

We were strict about Sundays too. If we needed work done on our homes, we agreed beforehand that the workmen would not work on Sundays. That was the condition for employing them.

My working life lasted from the age of fourteen to the age of sixty-nine. My first job was for a coal merchant's office. I collected payment for the coal that had been delivered to people's homes, and made sure there was none left on the pavement. I was not always a popular visitor! I worked for British Rail, from being sixteen up to the day of my retirement. For a little while I was a parcel porter, and then a porter, but for fifty-three years I worked as a shunter. It was hard work and we were given special clothing to protect us from bad weather. I worked near to Sheffield.

I can remember seeing my first car and my first tram. I was married to my first wife for forty years. After she died I married Doris, who was an old friend, and we have been married now for thirty-three years. We lived in a council house near our present home until we could not manage anymore. We chose the nursing home where we have now lived for two years because it is a Christian home. It makes all the difference in the world to be living in a Christian place. We are very contented here. We would not want to be anywhere else. We live quietly in our room. We don't go downstairs now. We take our meals in our room. We were struggling to see and hear the TV so we got rid of it. My son visits twice a week and we enjoy talking with the staff who work here.

### My Friend

Long years have passed since first I met
My Saviour on this road
When I just then with deep regret
Gave him my heavy load

I didn't know him very well
But knew that he was kind
I knew he had that special love
For which my heart had pined

So up the hill and down the dale
He travels life with me
He'll never falter never fail
Until his face I see

When I look back upon this life
My folly and my sin
How could he die upon that cross
My selfish heart to win

How could I ever doubt his love
When through this vale of tears
He's watched me from his home above
Throughout these struggling years

Betty Maclean

## BISHOP LESSLIE NEWBIGIN

As I have tried to look back over my life – and I have done this in writing an autobiography – my first overwhelming impression has been one of wonder and thanksgiving at the ways in which God has led me quite other than those I had expected or planned. The second is that of penitence as I reflect upon things which at the time seemed praiseworthy, but are now seen to be matters for penitence and for a revision and reformation of my style of living and thinking. The third matter concerns things in which I was involved and where the results have been quite different from what I hoped and planned for. Here I have many perplexities, for in some of the major decisions I have taken, though they were the right decisions, the results have been quite other than those I hoped for. I can only try to deal with this on the basis of my faith that God is the God who calls the things that are not as though they were and raises the dead to life.

## CLARE CLUCAS

I feel strongly that those of us who are older must try not to dwell overmuch on the past, but look to the future. On the other hand, there is a place for treasuring memories. I have written down things that I recall from the past for the benefit and interest of my children. I keep a file to which I add details of things my parents said about their childhood. I also spend time researching earlier generations of the family, finding photographs and records to add to the file. It is an absorbing and pleasurable hobby.

Another aspect of my approach to the past is to try to dispose of unwanted clutter. By this I mean not only possessions I no longer need, but also attitudes which are unhealthy, such as prejudices, for example, towards younger generations. I feel also that it has been important to make a clear will, specifying which of our belongings we would wish the various members of our family to inherit. In my case, this has meant giving instructions about my jewellery, so that more remote relatives and dear friends are not left out.

## PAUL TOURNIER

### Acceptance

Each of us dies a little in the death of those we love, and there is a part of our lives which ever afterwards we feel to be incomplete.

There are things we wish we had said, things we should have liked forgiveness for, things we should like to have heard, comfort we should like to have received . . .

But the pain of unfulfilment is not felt only in exceptional and dramatic situations. It is a daily occurrence. We die a little every day in all the things we leave uncompleted. All work is a beginning which does not really finish . . . . The unfulfilled is always felt as a failure. And when our children grow up, which of us can think about them with the clear conscience of parents who have fulfilled their mission? . . .

Jesus himself knew this pain, for, as St Paul says, he did not take advantage of his divinity in order to escape any human suffering (Philippians 2.6–7) . . . .

Look at those disgruntled old people who cannot accept their failing strength. Many of them have been no better at accepting their active lives before retirement. They grumbled then about their work and the responsibilities they had to shoulder; and they regretted their childhood, which also they had frequently not accepted either. The free and convinced consent that life demands of the old is not some exceptional burden that is laid on them alone – it is a universal law. A single 'Yes!' goes through the whole of life. It is successively 'Yes!' to childhood, to youth, to adult life, to old age, and finally 'Yes!' to death.

> From Paul Tournier's *Learning to Grow Old* (English
> tr., SCM press 1972).


## REG WYATT

As to looking back over my achievements, it is something I am rarely disposed to do, because current projects and interests seem much more worthy of time and attention than dwelling on the past. I suppose learning from the past has been an ongoing and contemporaneous assessment rather than a grand review at retirement of achievements or failures at each stage of life. It is not surprising, therefore, that I rarely dwell on memories or cherish times of love and happiness in the past.

Nevertheless, occasionally I find it rewarding to recall how much God, in his love and concern for me, particularly through salvation, has achieved in me by way of sanctification. I remember what sort of person I was, and then ask myself what sort of person I would be now were it not for the Lord's saving grace in my life. This leads me to praise him, and I am thankful that he intends to complete the task!

Sometimes, in sadder moments, failures and disappointments come to mind. My reaction to these occasions is immediately to dismiss the thoughts: to put away any regret and let the past remain in the past. I cannot turn the clock back, the failures cannot be eradicated; hopefully I have learned from the mistakes. I rarely dwell on my modest achievements, because I cannot rest on my laurels; it is not profitable. There is much satisfaction in what I am doing now, and I have much to look forward to.

## JOHN LIDBETTER

I was born in 1900, left school, where I was top boy, to start work at thirteen and a half. As a telegraph messenger I attended evening classes to prepare me for progress in the Civil Service.

When I was eighteen I was called to the Colours and served in the Royal Naval Volunteer Reserve until the end of the Great War. I served a short period as a postman and then took up my job as a sorter. I took a further examination for a clerical post and started as a clerical officer in the Ministry of Labour in August 1928.

My parents were godly people and I was brought up in a Christian home. I was baptized and received into the fellowship of the church when I was fourteen, but no story of my life would be complete or meaningful without reference to the spiritual crisis I experienced in 1924. Until that year my life had been fully occupied with sport and athletics. I had represented my office at cricket, football, tennis and running on the track. But on Maundy Thursday 1924, the crisis came in the form of a challenge from God. I was present at the funeral of a young friend who had been killed in a motor cycle accident while he was on God's service. The challenge that came to me was 'Why was this useful life taken and my useless life spared?' It was the turning point in my life. The next day was Good Friday and I was due to play football in the final for the Westminster Charity Cup. We lost the Cup and after the game I gave away my football gear, running spikes and all the paraphernalia of competitive sport. I had burned my boats! There was no return.

But a new life opened for me and I determined that I would be no less enthusiastic in serving the Lord Jesus Christ than I had been seeking my own pleasure. I gave my time to Bible study and fellowship with other Christians in their activities. My wife shared in all this change of lifestyle and our home became an open house for the Lord's people.

As Christian activities increased I found there was not time for a full-time job as well. I therefore retired from the Civil Service in 1961 to take responsibility for the work of Emmaus Bible School in the North of England. I was also an elder in my local church, and fully engaged in its ministry.

Having retired from secular employment I found increasing opportunities for Christian work. I became the honorary chaplain to a boys' public school in North Wales. This involved preaching on Sundays and general pastoral care of the boys and staff. I became a member of the Gideons International, serving with the North Wales branch, and I was able to help with the presentation of

New Testaments to schoolchildren, nurses, the police force and local hotels.

After six happy years of retirement, my wife suffered a severe stroke and for more than two years, until her death in 1970, she was my main concern. In the course of time I remarried and moved to Hendon, London, where my second wife lived. My membership of the Gideons was transferred to the North London branch where there was plenty of work to be done for the Lord. The work of visiting schools, hospitals and hotels gave opportunities to introduce people to the Bible and, in some instances, there was also scope for helping people in need of Christian comfort. I became an elder in the local church where I started an afternoon Bible class in the home of a member of the congregation. There was an old people's home quite near, where I had visited for the Gideons, and they were happy to have an afternoon service there once a fortnight, so I arranged this and took along some of the young people from the church to sing and talk to the residents. Beforehand we used to have a prayer meeting in our home followed by tea and this was a great opportunity to enjoy each other's company.

My wife was happy to support me in these activities. Retirement had brought me great opportunities for service and I am thankful to God that he gave me the good health which enabled me to lead such a rewarding life. I am now unable to do many of these things, but our home is still open for friends to visit and chat over a cup of tea. There is time for sharing happiness and heartache. May it be so until I am called home!

# 4

# Rediscovering Relationships

As we become older it can be that relationships come to mean more to us than they did in our younger lives. Despite the fact that old age is commonly believed to be a time of loneliness and isolation, of all the older people consulted in the British Gas survey, only one-fifth said that loneliness was a problem for them.

There are obstacles which prevent older people from enjoying friendship and intimacy. For one thing, they leave work which may have provided much of their social contact. Geographical mobility results in children and grandchildren living many miles away. Also, disability can render an individual housebound and reliant on others to visit them. Then there is the impact of bereavement. There is the sadness over the loss of a growing number of friends and relatives. But worst of all of course is the loss of a partner. It is somehow taken for granted that, because being widowed is an inevitable aspect of later life, older people naturally cope with its consequences. The experience can in truth be so devastating that it is common for the remaining spouse to outlive the other by a mere handful of weeks. Loneliness may not be unavoidable in later life, but it certainly can strike a person for periods of time.

Relationships change in retirement. For many there can

be some turbulence in married life as each partner adjusts to spending more time in the company of the other. Women speak of the frustration of the husband being around the house. Men say they feel the need to be out in order to keep from being 'under the wife's feet'. On the positive side, there can be a new sense of romance, of excitement, of mutual appreciation. There can be the joy of sharing activities previously undertaken without your partner, even apparently mundane tasks such as gardening, shopping and cleaning.

Another prominent relationship in retirement is the one many people have with their grandchildren. This can be a genuine highlight of later life. It is common for people to report that they find relating to their grandchildren easier and more rewarding than they ever found relationships with their own children. There is more time to develop closeness. There are none of the restrictions imposed by having to provide financial support. There is no disciplinary role. The bond is often mutually rewarding.

Perhaps one of the most fascinating insights to emerge from the British Gas survey of older people's attitudes was the finding that they were twice as likely to be 'enjoying life' if they claimed to have a lot of contact with younger people. Despite the tensions and misunderstandings between younger and older people, caused often by changes in society during the twentieth century, it is important to make sure that the generations do not retreat to their respective ghettos and lose contact with each other.

Older people undoubtedly give a great deal in relationships. They are found frequently caring for grandchildren whose parents are in paid employment, or looking after a disabled relative, or simply keeping an eye on a neighbour who needs support. Many elderly people have spent a lifetime developing skills of sensitivity and compassion in the way they relate to those they know.

## ELISABETH CHURCH

Behind him the lights of the Christmas tree threw shadows on his face. His dark eyes shone with happiness. Carefully I cut the cellophane and took time opening up the bright paper.

'What can this be?' I said, 'a lovely surprise I'm sure.'

I lifted his lovingly painted calendar out of its wrapping and put my arms round him for a hug.

Presents from grandchildren say so much. Time spent out of love. That element of surprise and the old truth that it is better to give than to receive.

Down the years how many such gifts have been made and given – models in clay or plasticine, tiny earrings or necklaces and many handmade birthday cards. Later the gifts become more sophisticated like the very beautiful real silk square handed to me by a medical student grandson and his sister. 'We knew you wear greens and browns, Zizz' (their name for me).

All these gifts are treasured – many sit on a shelf or little space for years and one is reluctant to part with them . . . .

Our twelve grandchildren are all different and yet a certain family likeness can be traced in them all. It is fascinating seeing the likeness in them to their own parents (our children), mannerisms too are so often family ones – sometimes as they grow up we see inherited gifts.

Now they range from twenty-nine down to seven years and the older ones are fanning out into the world and such a different world today.

It is a privilege when they come and want to talk. The secret is to listen, listen, listen. It is fatal to fire a lot of questions about their lives or friends. Wait and see what they tell you.

From *For Ever Jubilant: The Adventure of Ageing* by
Elisabeth Church (1993).

## BETTY MACLEAN

As far back as I can remember all I ever wanted to do was to be a wife and a mum. I had no great ambitions other than wanting a home and a family. I married young and had the first of my three children when I was only twenty years old. Things were often rough, but I was totally fulfilled. My family were spread over fifteen years, so I was fifty-seven when my youngest left home. During this time my first husband had passed away and I had remarried. Life was beginning to look up and we had started a small business, but after only one year my husband suffered a severe stroke, so again I had to take a step back and ask the Lord, where do I go from here?

I had nursed my first husband through four brain haemmorrhages, the first when I was just twenty-one. I have always helped a lot with my grandson who is a severe haemophiliac and also has hepatitis C, so I was no stranger to illness. But as I tried to come to terms with this latest blow, I realized that our retirement was going to be nothing like we had planned.

I prayed at this time as I have never prayed before. I saw that this situation was totally different from everything I had ever faced. It was going to affect both our lives, because Tom would need round-the-clock care. We had to build our lives around what we had left. The first thing I did was to borrow some books from the library to learn as much as I could about what had happened to both the body and the mind. I realized at this point how little I knew, and also how much caring was going to change my life. I will never say it has been easy, but I can say it has been rewarding. There have been many times when I have felt like giving up and at times I have wondered why we were only allowed two years of marriage.

But we have been blessed with some wonderful friends and a good family. There has always been a shoulder to cry on. We prayed a lot together as we started to plan our new life. The first thing I had to do was to learn to drive. So, at the age of fifty-two, I had to have lessons. These were going to be expensive and our bank balance was not in the best of health as we had only just begun to find our feet in the business. Right from the start, though, we saw the hand of God in everything we had to do. Tom and I looked after two dear old ladies who lived next door and had gone into hospital when Tom took ill. The older one had died, and her niece came round to give me a cheque. Although I tried to refuse it, she insisted I take it as she said it was for the kindness we had shown to them both. The cheque was for one hundred pounds, more than enough for my driving lessons. I felt that this must be from the Lord, as we are not in the habit of receiving such large sums of money.

After I passed my test, we spent the summers going on drives and picnicking in the car, as Tom was unable to walk. We even managed several little holidays. After a few years I was granted some help at home, which gave me some time to myself, but sadly two years ago Tom had to have both his legs amputated because of gangrene. Through all this, I have seen Tom grow spiritually and, although he spends a lot of his time in bed, he never complains and constantly witnesses to God's goodness.

It is now over seven years since Tom had his stroke and I have learned so much. I feel I can understand the less fortunate so much better. We still lead a very full life. Our home is always full because we say our home and car belong to the Lord and try to use them for his glory. Thanks to the help I get, I still have time to spend with my grandchildren. Two of them are in their teens now, so I feel very privileged that they still want to be with me.

I have also started writing poems again. This is something I have always done for my own amusement, but I have now offered them for publication and have had three printed and an invitation to submit two more. This again is an answer to prayer, because, as I get older, I am finding it more difficult to take Tom out. I prayed that the Lord would give me some other way to witness, and the publishers that have accepted my work are Christian-based.

So as I look forward to our remaining years, I thank God for each day we have together, for Tom's love and patience, for my children and my friends, and for a million and one other things, but most of all for giving me eternal life and for helping me through this one.

### FATHER MICHAEL

I am very lucky to be in this Community now that I am growing old. Luckier than my sister's poor husband, now that he is left. I think widowers are more to be pitied than widows these days. They are lost. He will feel lost. Whatever happens, you cannot be lost in the Community. You don't even retire because if you only go to chapel you continue to give and take your share there. A few days ago I returned to choir-practice. I'd given it up because the choir-school was so dreadfully cold – it has an outside wall! I'm not much good at singing now but every voice contributes something. In a community one is always useful. There is no one here who is not useful. We stay useful and see that we are kept useful and we know that death alone can end our usefulness. It has to do with keeping the Christian pattern. Most Christians have a pattern of prayer and know that to keep it when you are old is a great help generally. It is harder – hard – if you are on your own, of course, and not in a community.

From Ronald Blythe's *The View in Winter: Reflections on Old Age* (Penguin Books 1981).

### REG WYATT

Until seven years ago I had no expectation of being married in retirement, after separating from my first wife in 1982.

Being a bachelor again for about seven years might have
been expected to prejudice a successful second marriage.
However, my new marriage has been happy despite occasional stresses and strains. The fact that we were both on
our own for some years before marrying explains why
we both need our own 'space' and times of solitude. Our
difficulty is managing this need effectively.

Fortunately, we have several interests in common, so
there is much to share. Vacations together are, not surprisingly, a compromise, for I prefer an active holiday and
my wife a passive one. I love to stride the hills and she
loves to sit quietly, reading or doing a crossword.

We have no grandchildren and do not regret this, so it
is no problem for us. We have three adult offspring between
us, two some distance away, one quite near. We do not live
in each other's pockets, by mutual consent. We do not
hold on to them, they do not cling to us. But we commu-
nicate regularly and visit periodically. As parents we
believe that our children have their own lives to lead, their
own decisions to make. We do not interfere or give advice
unless asked. However, we are ready to help out practically
or financially when necessary.

I personally do not make friends, in the fullest sense of
the word, easily. I am very self-contained and perhaps lacking in warmth. I find it difficult to get close to people.
However, that's my nature.


## PHYLLIS WISEMAN

My life has included a number of changes, so it would be
natural to assume that I find change easy, but the reverse
is true.

I spent the first ten years of my working life, over the
war years, as a bank clerk. During that time I felt called
to missionary work but did not pass the medical. I then
decided to push the door which attracted me, namely work
in a residential children's home. After training, which

included practical experiences in Hertfordshire and Cheshire, I finally spent most of my twenty odd years in Norfolk as a housemother. When this home closed, I moved to Hertfordshire with my family group and, while there, it became obvious over a two-year period and with prayer that I needed to return home to look after my mother. I rejected a friend's suggestion that I should train as a teacher.

After pursuing other avenues, I finally accepted that my friend's advice was from the Lord. The college was conveniently in the next road to my home and even more miraculously I was accepted on a course for junior school teaching which would be completed *the year the college closed*. It was, of course, a great wrench to leave my group of children who could not be expected to understand. For me, it was an experience similar to bereavement, but the need to work hard academically helped; my mind was kept busy – the Master's hand at work again.

I passed my course which specialized in religious education and at the end was accepted by the Essex Education Committee. Teachers' places were being cut back and I was in my early fifties. After two temporary jobs, I was finally appointed to a special unit at Stansted which became a permanent post when a special school opened there.

Although not trained to specialize in the needs of severely mentally disabled children, I enjoyed my work. The caring side of it resembled my previous role. It also required less time in preparation and marking, giving me more time for my mother, now a widow. I retired when I was sixty.

My mother needed more of my time, but what did God want me to do as well? I tried Meals on Wheels, but that did not seem to be the answer. I happened to be visiting a young married woman and she told me about her work with the Citizens' Advice Bureau. I felt immediately that this was God's directing. I found the training and work quite tough due to my lack of confidence, but God had opened the door and I would stick it out until he closed it. Eventually I overcame my anxieties and enjoyed being of help to people. It was therefore with some regret that I gave up the work at sixty-five years of age because my mother needed me.

During my time at home I had taken on various jobs in the Baptist Church. I was a deacon and prepared the Holy Communion. I occasionally addressed women's meetings or took a Bible study. Since my mother's death, when I was sixty-nine, I have continued these tasks. I run a tape ministry for older ladies in my home one morning a week, and am also a pastoral group key person.

As I look back over the years it is good to see God's hand at work in so many ways, preparing me for what was to come. Listening to my teenagers in the early days has helped me in listening to adults. Housegroups have grown out of earlier attempts with a youngsters' Sunday evening group in Norfolk and a staff group in Hertfordshire. There have been hard lessons, too, to learn about myself – fortunately God only challenges us in small bites and is alongside to help.

If I were to criticize myself on my allocation of time now, I would say I am too tied to Christian activities and therefore not obeying the Lord's command to 'go'. Maybe I will try to follow the ambition I have to paint. When we are working it is accepted we are not available, but that is not the case when we are retired; there is more pressure from without and within to become involved. However, the plus side is that we all enjoy being needed.

I still have contact with some of the children I brought up, and on my seventieth birthday we had a get-together for staff and old boys and girls. Judging by the noise, it was enjoyed by all! So, although I have never married, I still see some of my 'grandchildren' and life has been very fulfilling in many ways.

## PAM WYATT

On several occasions I had read that retirement came near the top of any list of events which produced stress, and I faced the prospect of my husband's retirement with very mixed feelings. Part of me rejoiced with him as he looked forward to the freedom it would bring, and I welcomed the opportunity to spend more time with him. We shared many interests, including a passion for gardening and the countryside, and the future should have looked bright.

There was, however, another part of me which was secretly apprehensive about the possibility of losing the freedom to choose how I spent my time, and I was fairly certain that my nicely organized life was about to vanish. I felt selfish and guilty about this and found it difficult to discuss my feelings with anyone, even Reg or my prayer partner. However, we did talk to some extent about the changes we thought retirement would make in both our lives and, as Christians, believed that with the Lord's help we would overcome any relationship difficulties which might arise.

Looking back over the last four years, I now realize how unprepared we were to face such a major change in our lives, coming as it did at a time when we were still learning to live with another person after many years on our own. How much we would have benefited from talking to other retired couples.

Reg went on a pre-retirement residential course arranged by his employers, and this was valuable in providing useful information about financial matters and giving advice about developing interests and hobbies. There was, apparently, no discussion about how couples needed to look at the future together, and no suggestion that spouses might accompany their partners on the course.

It also occurs to me now that I have never seen an advertisement for a Christian retirement preparation course, either locally or in a Christian newspaper or magazine, and this would have been particularly useful.

Retirement is a frequent topic of conversation among our friends and relatives, many of whom are now in their late fifties or older. I have begun to realize, when talking with other women, that I was not alone in feeling as I did before Reg retired. I am also now more aware of the fears and problems which men encounter at this time in their lives. As on so many other occasions, I wish I had known then what I know now!

Needless to say, many of my fears were unjustified, but it has not always been easy. We have had to be willing to learn from our mistakes and, above all, to 'prefer each other in love'.

On the practical side, we have learned how to share responsibilities and chores as well as pleasures and, important for both of us, to allow each other a measure of personal space. This means that we have separate as well as joint friendships and a recognition that each of us has a need for times of solitude as well as enjoying each other's company.

Although we both wish that we had had a better preparation for retirement, we recognize that our Christian faith has been the most important factor in enabling us to work through the difficult patches together, and we praise the Lord for the joy he has brought us and the lessons we have learned.

As for relationships with our children, it is interesting to look back over the years and recognize the various stages we have been through. In the beginning there is the delight in the experience of parenthood, and an unfamiliar compulsion to protect and cherish. At the same time there is the realization that life will never be the same again. The sleepless nights and other problems associated with the early years can sometimes temporarily affect the relationship, but the bonding between parent and child is usually strong enough to help both of you to survive even the most difficult times.

As the years go by, the relationship changes as the individuality of the child begins to emerge, and there comes a time when we have to come to terms with the fact that the fledgling will need to test his wings and fly off into the world on his own. 'Don't fuss, Mum!' becomes a familiar phrase, and we have to trust in God and let them go.

Now that our children have lived independent lives for some years, the relationship has changed again. It is always good to see them, and while we enjoy their company, we do not live in each other's pockets. We are there for them if they need us, but it is just as true to say that they are also there for us. We now meet on equal terms, even though our lives and beliefs may be quite different, and we have learned not to have any expectations of them other than those they have for themselves.

## BISHOP LESSLIE NEWBIGIN

One of the great blessings of old age has been the opportunity to come to know our children and grandchildren. Because of long periods of living abroad we had not really got to know them. But now we live in London, where three of our four children with their families are near neighbours, we are coming to know and understand them in a way that we never could before. We are both learning much from this experience.

## DR BILL YOUNG

Having passed my 'sell-by' date (according to biblical reckoning) some ten years ago, my thoughts on ageing are no longer theoretical. I read recently in the *British Medical Journal* that exercising the mind may help in preventing its deterioration. I confess it was not with that in mind that, when I was retiring from general practice, I considered trying my hand at writing. Looking back, I think it was a short bout of flu and reading *All Creatures Great and Small* by James Herriot that started me thinking, 'I believe I could do something like that – from the medical angle'. I believe it may have helped my mind, but whether it did or not it was certainly fun and, though five books later with around 80,000 copies sold I am very little better off, I still think it was worth trying.

Ageing, with inevitable retirement, can be a difficult time. As a GP, one minute you are in a position of some authority, people are coming to you expecting help, your days are organized to the hilt, and the next minute you are out on your ear – one of a crowd, with perhaps a fishing rod from your staff and a few kind letters from former patients to show for all those years. (Mind you, it is just as well to keep out of places like supermarkets or you may find an elderly former patient who insists on showing you her swollen leg in one of the aisles!)

One thing you have plenty of in retirement is TIME. Time to use and not just to fill. Publishing a book can take up a lot of it (perhaps two years per book). It also takes a lot of patience and a long-suffering wife. But I still 'hae ma doots' about this business of preventing mental deterioration. I find numerous signs of it in myself – like going to the kitchen and forgetting why. It is of some comfort to know that a great writer like G. K. Chesterton is reputed to have sent a telegram to his wife saying, 'I am in Birmingham. Why?'

Yet another writer, Charles Swindoll, in his book *Strengthening Your Grip, on . . . Integrity, Prayer, Godliness, Evangelism . . .* has written a chapter on ageing. He enumerates some of the signs of it:

> You sit down in a rocking chair and can't get it started . . . the little grey-haired lady you help across the street is your wife . . . everything hurts and what doesn't hurt doesn't work . . . you sink your teeth into a juicy steak and they stay there . . . you watch a pretty girl go by and your pacemaker makes the garage door open.

The best medicine for ageing and the rest of life that I have found is accepting the love and forgiveness of the great physician, Jesus Christ. I once discovered that a patient who had come regularly for repeats of the medicine I had prescribed, had accumulated a cupboard full of it in her home. Some of us are a bit like that. Maybe we go to church, maybe we listen to 'Songs of Praise' or services on the radio, but we never 'take the medicine'.

I was especially glad of it when my dear wife, Betty, died. We had been married for nearly fifty-one years. In spite of the kindness of my family, I was undoubtedly lonely. But I found the presence of Jesus increasingly real. I could not wish her back; her last months had been ones of great suffering. I thought, well, it will only be a matter of time before I go and join her. God had other ideas. Some time passed and I crossed paths with another lady, Flora. A friendship sprang up and I began to feel that we might join forces. To be honest, it took me a matter of three weeks to reach this conclusion! She was not so sure! In fact, she said, 'But you hardly know me!' I said, 'I was a doctor for over fifty years and if I can't diagnose some-one in three weeks, I can't have been much good!'

Our families, all twenty-seven members of them, agreed with me, so Flora gave in. Today is the third anniversary of our wedding. It seems that good marriages *are* worth repeating.

I should stop there, but even though I am retired, I cannot stop giving advice, so here is a little more.

On retiring, don't move to the 'Shangri-la' of your honeymoon. It is probably a long way from your family and they will be busy, if you are not, and you may not see much of them. (Again, like some doctors, we did not take our own medicine – we moved. But we moved next door to our daughter).

Which leads me to my next bit of advice. It is from the Bible: 'Seldom set foot in your neighbour's house, too much of you and he will hate you' (Proverbs 25.17). I doubt whether our particular neighbours would actually 'hate' us, but they would find it very trying! Lastly, to anyone, young or ageing, if you want to be truly happy, I would say, read your Bible (preferably a modern version) and pray every day, and keep a sense of humour. Learn to laugh at yourself. It saves other people having to laugh at you!

## CLARE CLUCAS

In some senses, my attitude towards relationships has not altered in retirement. My family have always been the most important part of my life and continue to be. I am close to all three of my children and my six grandchildren who range in age from twenty-five down to eight. Although my children do not live close, they are very caring and supportive. When I was in hospital recently, one of my sons took leave from work in order to be with my husband.

I have needed to learn how to relate to my grandchildren as they have grown older. I enjoy their company greatly, but have realized that it is vital to be prepared to listen without offering advice. I hope I am good at keeping silent when I don't readily approve of their lifestyles. In particular, it is difficult to see a grandchild living with her boyfriend, as is normal now. Even when sorely tempted, I refrain from interfering in the upbringing of my grandchildren! I also feel it is important to be sensitive in conversation and talk about the past with grandchildren only if they seem genuinely interested.

I have close relationships in other contexts too. My voluntary caring group is like a family, supporting each other when times are hard. I have good friendship from amongst residents in the group of twelve flats where we live. I know they would be willing to help out if it was ever necessary. Also my minister and friends at church are supportive. I cannot speak too highly of the care and prayerful support we both receive.

# 5

# Coping with Loss

Some would view loss as the essence of old age. The contributors to this book tell a different story, and so only this chapter and the next focus on the sadness and challenges of later life.

Loss in retirement takes many forms. Perhaps the earliest dimensions become apparent with the process of retiring itself, with the loss of status and income that can also result. Leaving behind a career which may have brought tremendous satisfaction and reward is far from easy for some people (though for others there is a sense of relief). Owning the title 'pensioner' can feel like becoming a nobody. Another source of grief may be the physical decline ageing brings. We perhaps mourn the passing of the fitness and vitality of earlier years as they are replaced by waning energy levels and the onset of aches and stiffness in the joints. Many people bemoan the passing of their looks and are unhappy with their appearance in the mirror: 'Can that really be me?'

A further aspect of loss is the regret and sadness a person can feel over the past. Opportunities missed, failings, broken relationships and unfulfilled ambitions can return to haunt us. What went before cannot be changed, history cannot be rewritten. Dreams for the future feel pointless, too, as they will never come to fruition.

Then comes the series of losses which perhaps hurt the

most. There are the deaths of many who were loved and formed a vital part of life. There may be a succession of friends to whom to say goodbye. And amongst the relatives who go may be that special person to whom we were joined in marriage so many years before. It is hard to imagine how it can be possible to find a new way of living when your existence has been so closely entwined with that of a lost loved one over the course of many years. In Christian marriage two become one. Returning to singleness can feel strange and unpleasant.

Strangely, though, older people are expected to possess the resources with which to handle this succession of losses and the grief they provoke. Because loss is a natural component of old age, we assume that older people are somehow prepared to meet its reality with a store of inner strength. And it is also taken for granted that feeling sad is part and parcel of being older. Whereas when younger people exhibit symptoms of depression, action is taken to ensure that they regain their equilibrium, older people are very often left to suffer with no help. In fact, there are a great many retired people suffering unnecessarily from depressive illness.

Despite becoming familiar with the experience of loss, many older people are remarkably positive in their outlook; having reached a measure of acceptance they are determined to find things for which to thank God. Many transform their personal suffering into a source of benefit to others. They exercise a calm forbearance, a gentle kindness and an empathy which can bring blessing to those around them.

The accounts of older people featured in this book may give the impression that life is far from fair. There are individuals for whom later life is a sequence of devastating blows. For others, on the other hand, retirement is packed with halcyon days. The Christian community has a responsibility to offer support and friendship to older people whose lives are filled with a sense of loss and desolation.

## PAM WYATT

A few years before she died at the age of eighty-two, my mother spoke to me of how isolated she felt. I found this difficult to understand as she had frequent visits from her children and grandchildren. She was on good terms with her neighbours and, being very active for her age, enjoyed various hobbies which brought her into contact with many people. She had always found it easy to make friends and, even though my father had died a few years before, in many ways this had brought her a new freedom.

As I get older myself, I am beginning to understand that solitude takes many forms and does not necessarily always mean absence of people. I have recently lost one or two lifelong friends and, although there are many left, I am more easily able to see what she was saying. She had explained that there was virtually nobody left in her life who knew her when she was a young girl or in the early years of marriage. When I was younger I had enjoyed hearing about her schooldays, her much-mourned first love and the hopes and disappointments of those far-away years. Now, although she could reminisce, there was no-one left to whom she could say, 'Do you remember . . . ?', and an important part of her life had gone for ever. She was beginning to feel isolated and unnecessary in a world which put a great deal of emphasis on youth.

It was round about this time that she started to attend church regularly after an absence of nearly sixty years, and she was subsequently confirmed. After her death, I found little jottings in the back of her prayer book which spoke of the unexpected joy she had found in coming to know the Lord and becoming a part of a Christian family as well as a human one. Never again did I hear her say that she felt isolated, and I am sure that she found a new fulfilment in a church where she was aware of being valued, used and loved.

The church was packed for her funeral.

### Bereavement

Dark place,
Where, vulnerable, alone,
We lick the wounds of loss.

Wise friends say little
But hold us in their love,
And listen.

There are no guarantees,
Only reports from those
Who've been there,
That there is hope,
And life persists.

                                    Ann Lewin


## LYDIA DUCKWORTH

I am ninety-two and I have lived at Highfield House residential home for seven years now. No one wants to give up their home, but you have to look at it a certain way, and realize that, if you cannot manage, you have no alternative but to go into a home. I found it hard to adjust at first to the selfishness and childishness of the other residents, who always put themselves first. I used to spend all my time downstairs, but a year or so ago I decided to stay in my room. There are three steps up to my room which the lift does not reach. I was finding them difficult to manage and did not like putting the staff to trouble.

Also, in the lounge most people are deaf so I was exhausted every evening after spending the day shouting. They also tended to fall asleep after breakfast. And there is one woman who, whilst she has her good points, dominates the TV. She tells other residents' visitors to be quiet whilst she is watching, whereas her guests interrupt other people's programmes. In my room I can watch whatever I like at the volume I choose. I also have plenty of visitors, so I never feel bored.

Now I find it hard to walk, I do get frustrated, but I try to think how fortunate I am in having my hearing and eyesight still. I get annoyed when I drop things and find it so difficult to pick them up.

Now I am no longer able to go out, I particularly miss visiting my sister's house and going to church. I used to love the Wednesday morning services, and would encourage other people to go. But I discovered that they were not given a welcome by the regulars. One lady whose baby was noisy during the service was so upset by the stares of the other people that she never returned. I love children.

Church was my life as a child. We had a father in a million who always took us to services and used to run the Sunday School. I remember when my brother and I were young our father sat us behind a pillar. He said that was where we were to sit until we were old enough to behave and be on view!

I have had a lot of trouble, though, so at times in my life I have lost my faith and wondered what my father would have said. I felt God ill-treated me, and took away all I had. I had an unhappy marriage. Then my only son, Frank, died at the age of fifty. I think it went back to an accident he had when he was three and which he was lucky to survive. His wife would not allow a post-mortem. Then two years later, my only grandchild, Ann, died of cancer at the age of twenty-four. My daughter-in-law then stopped visiting me. We had not been close, but had never had a cross word. Though she never asked my advice and would not visit me unless she was with Frank or Ann, I had always kept quiet about things she did that I did not like. I was heartbroken when she did not come to see me and then sent beautiful cards at Christmas and birthdays. I stopped sending cards and then she did too. She remarried a few years after Ann died. She lives near here, but we have no contact.

At first I was bitter against God. I felt I had nobody left. But I slowly started to see things differently. Frank and Ann had been so close, I realized that it would have

broken his heart if he had not died first. Then I told
myself, 'You ought to be glad, they are together now in
heaven.' I say my prayers now every night.

I think about my memories. That is all I have now. A
man down the corridor from me, who has also lived here
seven years, pops in to chat for twenty minutes several
times each day. We talk over old times, and, though he is
much younger than me, we share memories of poverty and
hardship. When I was just twelve I began work in a local
cotton mill. At thirteen I went full-time, starting at 6.00 am
and working a fifty-five-hour week. I was always a 'homebird'
so, when my youngest sister was born and I was fifteen, my
father arranged for me to be off work for six weeks to look
after my mum. I was happy working long hours to bring in
extra money for my parents. In the 1930s times were hard.
Unemployment was high and there was no social security.
It was piecework, you see, with no regular salary. During
the war I got on well because so many of the looms were
empty.

When I first married, at twenty-four, we lived with my
parents. When we had our own home, we needed to save
to pay for furniture and repairs to the house which was in
poor condition. My idea was to work hard and get on, but
my husband would not try. His mill was not as good as
ours – our boss had only the one mill. So when Frank was
only four months old I faced the humiliation of queueing
up each day outside the mill to see if there was any work
available. However much I tried, I was flogging a dead
horse. And they say that worry kills you!

We had so much hardship in those days. People now
don't know they are born. Right up to moving here I never
had hot running water in my house, and I had an outside
toilet too. My hair has never gone grey and the other residents cannot believe I don't treat it. It doesn't bother
me. I never think about my hair! I cannot understand why
people spend their money on trying to look younger.

Sometimes I say to myself, 'Why have you lived to be this age? What good are you doing?'

---

### A Meditation on Grief

There is a time for everything, and a season for every activity under heaven.

A time for giving birth, for dying, for planting, for reaping, for weeping, for laughing, for mourning, for dancing, for keeping, for throwing away;

A time to mourn is a time when we can bring to God our feelings, our grief reactions.

The shock and numbness, the tightening in the chest as though an iron hand is squeezing the heart when first we heard of the death of the one we loved.

We said, as Jesus did, 'Father take this cup from me, my cup is so full of hurt and tears it's just too much for me to hold.' It's too much to ask of me to say, as Jesus did, 'Yet not my will but yours be done' (Luke 22.42–3). Not my will but yours be done. When we are hurting we want so much for the hurt to be taken away. We deny the reality of our loss. After Jesus' arrest, Peter denied that he ever knew Jesus, three times, and went outside and wept. A time to weep.

Our denial can often make us quite angry. Jesus was fully human and he was angry. It is alright to give vent to anger. Jesus' anger drove out those selling in the temple (Luke 19.25). It is anger that makes us ask, 'How can a loving God allow me to suffer so?'

Can God really understand the times we stop and pause, or look out of the window and hope to see or hear our loved one?

Yes, God replies, 'While my son was a long way off I was filled with compassion for him. I ran to my son and threw my arms around him' (Luke 15.20). In this way I am also filled with compassion for you. I embrace you, and enfold you, my son and my daughter.

My human feelings were experienced through my son Jesus. 'I so loved you that I gave my one and only son' (John 3.16).

'You are healed by the punishment he suffered, made whole by the blows he received. I the Lord made the punishment fall on him' (Isaiah 53).

The release from the pain of our grief will come when we can accept that, 'Now the dwelling of God is with you and he will live with you and be your God. He will wipe away every tear from your eyes.' Acceptance is about acknowledging the feelings associated with our loss, expressing them and then being enabled by God to remember without the hurt.

We can never know fully, Lord, just what it cost you to live and die on this earth, but if the pain of our grief enables us to draw nearer to you, perhaps we will understand a little more.

Written for use in churches by Freda Moody,
herself retired.

## ELISABETH CHURCH

Inevitably as octogenarians we anticipate our earthly life coming to an end. This must be for us the last lap. It does not alarm us. We love life but must be realistic. We naturally wonder which of us will be left behind and try to imagine what it must be like. Even the thought of writing 'widow' or 'widower' instead of 'married' on various forms will seem strange. All our bereaved friends tell us that until you have been through the loss of your nearest and dearest you cannot possibly imagine what it must be like. We respect that.

How strange it will be not to hear the familiar call on entering the house, or the cheerful shout down the stairs, or the well-known footsteps, or the scrape of a chair, or the clatter of washing up dishes.

How strange at night not to put out a hand and feel the warm comfort and know the other is there.

We sometimes discuss it all. What we would like? cremation? funeral? thanksgiving? memorial service? ashes, scattered or buried? These are the outward considerations; important though they are, the real meaning of loss is far deeper. 'Our outward man perishes but the inner man is renewed.' The real him or me will go on to the great unknown and never die, we have been promised that, we shall meet again.

I shall want to give thanks for all the years together if I am left. A great hymn of thankfulness. And I hope I shall be able to accept. I hope tears will come, they are part of grieving and of healing.

We have reached a point in life when many of our friends and family have died. We miss them greatly and feel the gap they leave. It is wonderful how many have left a 'sweet savour'. We remember them with gladness for the quality of their lives.

I cannot possibly tell how bereavement will affect me. I can imagine bleak loneliness. I know I must keep turning to Christ.

From *For Ever Jubilant: The Adventure of Ageing* by Elisabeth Church (1993).

## MARY MOYES

My first experience of caring was when my mother-in-law came to live with us. She came at very short notice but responded quickly to rest, care and home-cooking. Each day she was able to walk further until eventually neighbours were able to set their watches by our two daily walks! I was offered day care which made it possible for me to speak at meetings, and Mother kept herself busy making wonderful things like teapot stands to give to relatives.

As my husband's illness worsened, Mother asked to move to a nursing home. I continued to do her washing and take her for walks. My husband, Kenneth, was no longer able to be pastor of a church, but he was able to produce five magazines of various types. Before long he was using a wheelchair, but we were able to go to church together and even take part in an Easter march of witness. He went to painting classes in a local school whilst I did the shopping and he especially enjoyed attending ecumenical services held locally. We seemed to make more and more Christian friends wherever we went. We went on holiday to a specially adapted house in Ross-on-Wye and enjoyed the daily minibus rides.

Kenneth and I even travelled to Greece and Turkey on the journeys of St Paul. Despite the risks, these were wonderful spiritual experiences which helped us greatly. Though my husband's body was decreasing, God gave strength for these travels. Eventually, however, he became virtually bedridden. He was always so grateful for the help he received and was able to raise his arm in worship. We joined hands to praise God together silently.

We had nurses and home helps, and a neighbour's girl encouraged Ken when he was downstairs, helping him to paint with watercolours. I continued speaking at meetings. The help we were given gradually increased as I became able to accept that we needed it.

My husband passed away peacefully in hospital and so many queued at the crematorium for the service of thanksgiving. I was surrounded by family throughout and friends and clergy of all denominations were present. The following year my mother also passed away in a nursing home.

I myself found before long that I needed two total hip replacements. I felt very much blessed that my recovery was both swift and complete, to the amazement of those around me. Afterwards, I felt my ministry deepened further still. I am kept very busy, co-ordinating voluntary groups, speaking at meetings and offering counselling. My family spoil me. My life seems to be full of valuable moments and well worth the living. The days are never long enough. Much of my retirement has been spent cycling to local communities, hoping to meet those who may wish to join the Torch Trust for the blind and partially-sighted. I visit members of the group in their homes, taking with me tapes of Christian singing. I do not feel that being so busy is a way of crowding out memories.

I look back over our married life and remember the work we shared in churches. Kenneth was in Burma during the war. When he returned he was advised that it would be medically unwise to work, but, Kenneth being Kenneth, he immediately found a job and finished training as a pastor. Rebuilding after the war was a difficult time. I remember feeling lonely. There was no furniture or clothing in the shops. On one occasion I unstitched a blue wool coat to make a warm siren suit for my son.

Many of my memories are of happy family times: outings with grandchildren, the joy of pet animals, shared jokes and all the joys of a large family. I rejoice that I am surrounded by a vast array of friends still, but always keep in mind that the nearest friend, the Lord, is always present.

From my work with Cruse Bereavement Counselling, I have come to realize that we each need time to deal with grief in our own way, coming to terms with loss gradually. In time we become ourselves again. There are times when I do cry, when I suddenly feel lonely, even in a big crowd. Emotions are funny things, but I love reading and am always writing letters.

# 6

# Living with Disability

Some of the recent discussions over rationing scarce National Health Service resources have been enlightening in what they imply about later life. The Queen Mother provoked a good deal of interest when she underwent a successful hip replacement operation at an undeniably advanced age, but elsewhere it has been argued that treatment of certain conditions in retired people is a waste of public funds.

Part of the fear of old age in the minds of young people has to do with a tendency to view it as being synonymous with decrepitude. Unfortunately, few people realize that only five per cent of the retired population are dependent enough to live in some kind of institution. And neither do older people report ill-health as a major problem. Of the British Gas survey pensioners, 78 per cent said their health was either 'very good' or 'fairly good'. Ill-health in retirement seems to be confined to a small period at the end of a person's life.

On the other hand, it would be absurd to believe that, given scientific advances, we could avoid mortality altogether. Researchers in the USA have made extravagant claims for their discoveries about the ageing process. Before long, they believe, we could be living to the age of 200. Improvements in health and diet, it is true, have led to dramatic improvements in life expectancy during the twentieth century. Fundamentally, however, we are mortal and the scientists can but postpone the inevitable.

As our bodies gradually wind down towards the end of our lives, we may notice we have a dwindling supply of energy. We no longer possess the stamina to accomplish tasks we managed with ease in our earlier years. Actual disabilities can make an unwelcome appearance. Especially common are complaints such as rheumatism and arthritis which reduce mobility. Problems more likely in old age are osteoporosis and strokes, heart conditions and reduced hearing and eyesight. The challenge is to learn to accept these limitations and discover new and fulfilling pastimes which accommodate them.

Talking with older people, certain fears emerge as common themes. Whilst death itself often holds no fear for the Christian, there is the anxiety that the process of dying will be long and drawn out. There is also, in many older people, a concern never to become a 'burden' to their children if they become frail. Perhaps most dreaded of all is the prospect of losing your mind, of falling prey to the ravages of Alzheimer's disease.

The reverse side of the coin of disability is the responsibility carried by many pensioners for the care of other elderly people who cannot manage on their own. It can be a rough adjustment to find one's plans for freedom and fulfilment in retirement shattered by the need to look after someone in need. Life for these elderly carers, however, and the disabled relatives for whom they care, need not be unremittingly gloomy. Given adequate support, from public and private sources, and a reasonable level of income, the quality of life of families with incapacitated members can be excellent.

The sequel to this tale of disability in later life is heartening. In the pages of this book, as in the lives of many frail elderly Christians, we discover the mystery of suffering. Within Christian discipleship it is very often the experience of weakness and dependency which brings us closest to

God's presence. It is as we are stripped of our self-sufficiency that we turn to Christ for the strengthening and endurance he offers. Through our pain we identify with his pain and with a suffering world. We draw closer to the Father heart of God. And so it is that from the most fragile and the sickest of elderly people there can radiate the compelling light of God's love. In their dependency they have found his grace to be sufficient.

> Lord God, pain is no stranger to me.
> It makes me testy and short tempered
> and I am not easy to live with.
> I get resentful of my illness
> especially when others, older than myself,
> appear to enjoy good health.
> They get out and about without handicap
> and my envy overflows.
>
> I pray for healing.
> I pray for the ability to accept my limitations
> and to trust in your power.
> To touch the hem of your garment
> is all I ask.
> Help me to see the forms your garment takes.
>
> If anything in my life,
> any build up of resentment
> and harboured hate,
> has brought me to where I am,
> then show it to me and release me from it.
>
> If my pain is part of yours
> and you need me as a witness
> to the strength which shows itself in weakness,
> then give me the patience, courage and fortitude
> I need.

From *A Pensioner's Prayer Book* by J. H. Speed
(John Paul the Preacher's Press 1981).

## ELISABETH CHURCH

Among half a century of old faded photographs there are highly glamorous ones of us by 'Lenare' at the time of our engagement. Clean complexions and thick wavy hair enhanced by the shining eyes. Living rapturously in the glorious present no thought of old age ever crossed our minds, and rightly so, for life is to be lived in its immediate context and the lovely times enjoyed to the full.

We took our health for granted. All the joys of hockey, tennis, swimming, fell-walking were ours. I never envisaged a time when physical powers would diminish. Of course with advancing age the machine will show wear and tear . . . .

Recently we were out walking in the New Forest. Howard's pedometer registered four miles and we were jubilant!

'Four is not bad is it?' we said, looking into each other's eyes. 'We could try five next time' and we opened the car door, threw our rucksacks and walking sticks in the car and sank thankfully into our seats reaching for the coffee flask.

'Four miles' I thought, recalling a day in Kenya when he and I had walked over the tail of the Elephant Mountain in the Aberdares. It was a total of twenty miles, up through the forest and bamboo in the mists of the moorland at 12,000 ft and then down to the vast plateau of the Kinangop.

Or again an unforgettable day in Skye swinging along the ten miles from Elgol to Torrin under the frowning heights of Blaven.

Walking over Dartmoor in my sixties and seventies meant leaping over leats and streams and landing safely on a bank or on stepping stones. With thumb-stick in hand we leapt with confidence because there

was still spring in our joints. Now the 'elastic' has
gone, no spring remains and we dare not trust a
jump – one can be such a nuisance with a broken
ankle!

Getting down to sit on the ground is difficult, but
far more difficult is getting up. We find the only way
is to roll over on to our knees and pull each other up.
Creaky bones have come to stay . . . .

All through these landmarks has been the need to
accept, accept. As each landmark of renunciation is
reached one seems to be cushioned against the blow
and it does not seem such a sacrifice at all.

> From *For Ever Jubilant: The Adventure of Ageing*
> by Elisabeth Church (1993).

## LORD LONGFORD

There are certain advantages and certain disadvantages
to being ninety. You get a lot of friendly comment.
The late Kingsley Martin, editor of the *New Statesman*,
said, 'What's gone wrong? No one is being nasty to
me any more. Aren't they frightened any longer?' In
fact, it is rather like winning a lottery. It is no virtue
of yours that you have achieved this so-called feat. On
the other hand, you do not get any money out of it.
Equally, no one imagines that you are better off as a
result. If you won the lottery people would come beg-
ging at your door and overwhelm you. But no one
thinks of a nonagenarian as having anything to spare.
So there are benefits and disadvantages.

I speak from what one might call a broadly human
point of view about these matters. We oldies have
certain physical and medical needs. However, on the
psychological side, it is worth asking ourselves what
old people do need. To start with, they need company.
Some of us are very lucky in that when we are old we

have a loving wife and so we are well looked after. Others are not so fortunate, or they may have lost their loving partner quite recently. One's heart goes out to them.

What can be done? The carers must try to provide something that they have lost. Activity and occupation are very much harder to provide for people as their disabilities grow, but an effort must be made. However, the particular point I want to make is about the need to give them what I call respectful help. As one gets older one's physical disabilities increase, although one likes to think that one becomes wiser and wiser. One may be mistaken in that, but there is no mistake in that one's physical disabilities increase.

The problem about old people is that they become very sensitive. It is difficult to know quite when to offer them help. I was brought up to offer my seat to a lady on the tube or anywhere else. Nowadays, if a lady offers her seat to me on the tube, I am in two minds about it, because I may be going only from Westminster to Sloane Square. In that case I would probably not accept it unless I was very tired. However, if I am going to Ealing or somewhere similarly far away, I gracefully accept the seat offered to me. That is one problem with the elderly: how to give them help? When you drop something on the floor people rush to pick it up. I fell down in the tube the other day and I think eight people tried to pull me to my feet. I could have got on very much better without them, but the intention was good. It is a question of how one provides tactful help.

Taken, with permission, from a speech delivered to the House of Lords on 6 December 1995 as part of a debate on long-term care for the elderly.

## PAM WYATT

The ageing process has happened so gradually that it was only when I was asked to contribute towards this book that I began to consider how much I had been affected by advancing years.

It is only now that I realize how much I have been making concessions to the wear and tear of over sixty years, and how my mobility and energy have decreased, particularly in the last two or three years.

For instance, not so long ago I would have welcomed the opportunity to spend an afternoon working in the garden and then gone off happily to do something else in the evening. Nowadays, two hours of weeding is enough, and the prospect of an evening at home is attractive. Where has all my former energy gone, particularly when I still feel so young inside?

Some of the joints in my body are painful and hands, neck and hip are becoming a problem, so I have had to resort to gadgets and tools to help the less physically-able. Pills and potions from my GP are a help for other parts of my body which do not function as well as they used to, but on the whole this sounds a lot worse than it actually is.

There are, naturally, some frustrations. I can no longer play the piano, and find I drop things more often than before. My energy is restricted, so I cannot spend as long as I like doing the things I enjoy (such as gardening), and have a good excuse not to do too much of the things I do not care for (such as cleaning). When we are on holiday my husband Reg has to go walking on his own if he wants more than a sedate ramble, and I do something less strenuous.

More worrying has been the increasing, and sometimes embarrassing, problem with failing powers of memory. It is no worse than that of others of my age, but my mother suffered from Alzheimer's disease towards the end of her life and I remember the burden this placed on my brother and sister-in-law. Although she could do virtually nothing for herself, she genuinely believed that she was coping as well as she did years before and was resistant to any suggestion that she needed full-time care. There is no reason to think that this will happen to me, and I know that having given this to the Lord I should be at peace about it, but this is not the first time I have given him a problem and then taken it back so that I can worry about it again. Help, Lord!

On the whole, however, I consider that I am still reasonably fit for my age and enjoy a fairly busy retirement. Despite the qualifications in the previous sentence, I am very much aware that I have much for which to thank God, not least for bringing me a husband with whom I can share these later, and best, years of my life.

A little over two years ago, we learned that Reg had cancer. All my own minor aches and pains became totally irrelevant. It only came to light by what some people might call 'chance', but we believe that it was the hand of God at work in our lives.

The waiting time between the tests and subsequent diagnosis was, in fact, quite short, but it seemed endless and we were very dependent on God to see us through this difficult period. Some verses from Psalm 145 were very comforting:

> The Lord is faithful to all his promises and loving towards all he has made. The Lord upholds all those who fall and lifts up all who are bowed down. (Psalm 145.13–14)

Two days after we learned about the cancer and the need for some weeks of debilitating treatment, we went to a mid-week service at church. The visiting preacher was an old friend of our fellowship and he and his wife had led a parish weekend-away for us a few years before. During a time of ministry following the sermon, we were both prayed for and Reg was anointed with oil. From that moment on, we were both filled with complete peace about the future and a certainty that whatever happened we were held in God's loving care. We must have said the words of the Grace many times over the years, but it was only then that we experienced 'the peace of God which passes all understanding' as an actual reality.

I realize that I have been using the word 'we' when speaking about Reg's illness, but the closeness of a good marriage means that when something like this happens to one partner, the other is as much involved and 'one flesh' takes on a new meaning.

We were helped in many ways while Reg was undergoing his radiotherapy treatment, but most important of all was the constant prayer support we received. We give thanks to God that all the tests have been negative for nearly two years now.

## REG WYATT

Disability for me amounts as yet only to decreasing physical strength and ability. Intermittent aches and pains, pulled muscles, strained ligaments (particularly in the lower back) are increasingly a nuisance. Heavy lifting is out and digging the garden, which does not do my back any good, has only recently been possible through the use of the 'claw', a new garden tool. I cannot sustain physical effort as long as I used to.

How does this affect me? Well, frustration first and foremost, because I have always enjoyed physical activities. I have never found it easy to sit around for any length of time. Thus, when I am out of circulation because of an injury, I become frustrated and restless. A lack of patience does not help. From time to time I have considered taking up drawing, painting and picture-framing as new channels of creativity. I have not got round to it yet, because the first two demand much time and patience, and the last requires instruction (I have yet to discover an evening class which teaches this). Perhaps the time will come when I will attempt these activities, but whilst I am able, gardening and the like will take up much of my time.

My wife Pamela does not enjoy robust health, although she is still very active. She loves gardening. I do experience heartache when she has bad days. But she is not one to be 'fussed', as she puts it, and so I do what is of practical help and allow her to rest quietly on her own.

## CATHERINE COOPER

Of course, if, and when, I get to the stage of being 'well stricken in years', I may not feel as energetic as I do now. Housebound, incapacitated, no convenient transport, so what can one still do as a believer? The classic answer seems to be, 'you can still pray'. Oh yes, but it would be nice to do a little more. It wouldn't be too difficult to do, say, at least one of the following each day:

- Invite a neighbour in for a cup of coffee.
- Write a letter to missionaries or someone who is lonely.
- Pick up the telephone . . . there is always someone who might appreciate a call.
- Say to myself . . . 'Don't just sit there . . . do something!'
- And above all, guard against becoming a 'prisoner of the box'.

The psalmist has much encouragement for us as older believers:

The righteous shall flourish like a palm tree . . .
They will still bear fruit in old age,
they will stay fresh and green,
proclaiming 'The Lord is upright . . . He is my Rock.'
(Psalm 92.12, 14–15)

Whatever 'bearing fruit' may mean in the context of this

verse, we can still bear fruit by proclaiming, 'The Lord is upright . . . He is my rock'.

With an increase in disabilities or loss of old friends, the days between the sunset and the stars is not a time perhaps to which one would look forward, but for me as a committed Christian the goal is clear. It is summed up in verses of a hymn written almost a hundred years ago, by Edith Gilling Cherry:

> We go in faith, our own great weakness feeling,
> And needing more each day Thy grace to know:
> Yet from our hearts a song of triumph pealing,
> 'We rest on Thee and in Thy Name we go.'
>
> We rest on Thee, our shield and our defender!
> Thine is the battle, Thine shall be the praise;
> When passing through the gates of pearly splendour,
> Victors, we rest with Thee through endless days.

# 7

# Growing into Spiritual Maturity

We never retire from being a disciple of Christ. The Bible is full of encouragement towards faith which develops and grows throughout the course of life. One biblical image is of the athlete 'pressing on' towards the goal and coming nearer and nearer to the kingdom of God. Older people find no justification for 'taking it easy' in the spiritual realm. This means that, instead of neglecting the insights of older Christians, we should be turning to them for advice and understanding. Many have walked with God through a lifetime and known his presence in the sorrowful and the joyful times alike. Unfortunately, this is not always reflected in the organization of church affairs, which is very often both under the control of younger people and designed to attract them.

Older people's preferences do differ from those of younger people. They often desire a more contemplative form of worship. Older people's devotional lives also develop. With later life comes a more reflective approach to faith, and the realization that 'being' is more important than 'doing' in our relationship with God. Finbarr Lynch, in an article in *The Way* (April 1996), says that prayer comes more naturally in later life: 'Prayer is no longer a compartment; it is a dimension, a climate, an atmosphere, a gift of awareness.' This is not to say, however, as is often presumed, that prayer is the only rightful ministry of the older Christian. Such an attitude often meets with frustration and disappointment on the part of retired people who wish to remain active in God's service.

People who grow old happily begin to see God in different ways. In place of the sober, severe father figure who applies rules and sanctions, there is a growing awareness of God's compassion, from which grows a willingness to accept diversity and a tolerance of ambiguity in expressing faith. Faith is seen as a mystery to be explored. Perhaps this broader understanding of faith and of the world in all its complexities is part of the 'wisdom' which the Bible associates with old age.

There is a fear within some Christians that later life will bring a loss of mental faculties which will impede their ability to relate to God. Faith, though, does not reside in the intellect. Even those with advanced dementia can be encouraged to continue worshipping. Many can be helped to take part in services through the use of favourite hymns and prayers, and familiar Bible readings. Communion can also mean a great deal to confused elderly people.

The case of the confused older person highlights the essential truth about the Christian faith. As David Wainwright affirms in this chapter, it is not what we are able to do in our Christian lives which holds ultimate value, but who we are. And our identity is shaped by God's act of love and saving grace. No matter what degree of frailty we face, our status is unchanged. Our primary duty is to become more Christ-like, whether in active service or passive infirmity. The wonder of the Christian pilgrimage is the truth that some of the most elderly and frail members of the Christian community can inspire others with conviction; because they can almost reach out and touch their Lord, their lives reflect powerfully his love and his radiance.

I am growing old
and still
I believe in God
more and more.
I don't know why
as hurt happens,
troubles never cease,
bringing opportunities for my growth,
fulfilling the hidden plan
God gave when I was born,
Promising his love for me.

Sue Norris

### CATHERINE COOPER

Last year I read a little book (the title eludes me) written about fifty years ago by a man named Henry Drummond, in which he said,

> The Jewish people regarded old age as being in three stages:
>
> 1) from 60 to 70 years . . . the commencement of old age
> 2) from 70 to 80 years . . . the 'hoary headed age'
> 3) from 80 years onwards . . . well stricken in years.

I belong in the second category! Jews held old age in respect and honour. The Mosaic law says: 'Rise in the presence of the aged, show respect for the elderly' (Leviticus 19.32). Sadly the cult of youth seems to have replaced respect and reverence for old age.

In the church to which my husband and I belong there is a gentleman's agreement that one retires from major responsibilities, for example, the diaconate, at the age of seventy. Of course, our gifts and responsibilities must be different as we get older. Health, mobility, and particularly staying power are all inclined to degenerate. And the little grey cells do keep dropping off!

However, I do not find any suggestion of retirement in the Bible. We may retire from secular work, but we should never retire from his work. As one of our family (aged forty) put it, 'Christians never retire. They go on till they drop'!

Many years ago, I well remember our youngest daughter coming home from school, frustrated and tearful, and flinging her schoolbag down in the hall crying, 'Ever felt unwanted?' Sometimes we can get this feeling too, that we are old, unwanted, redundant and unimportant. But of one thing we can be quite sure; the older generation is important to God. He says,

> Even to your old age and grey hairs
> I am he, I am he who will sustain you.
> I have made you and I will carry you.
> I will sustain and I will rescue you. (Isaiah 46.4)

And again, when the apostle Paul wrote to the Corinthian Church, he said, 'We do not lose heart. Though outwardly we are wasting away, yet inwardly we are being renewed day by day.'

So we are promised by God that he will sustain us, carry us, rescue and renew us. Although we change in many ways as our years increase, God's care for us is unchanging. He promises: 'Never will I leave you; never will I forsake you' (Hebrews 13.5). These promises I firmly believe.

Am I just growing older, or am I growing into more spiritual maturity as I grow older? I hope I am. There is certainly more time for prayer, especially intercessory prayer. I can pray about the events of the day, about people I have met, about letters received and written, and plans for the week. Then, too, Bible study can be leisurely and unhurried. There is more time for lending a listening ear, and perhaps visiting those not so fortunate as myself. I should be doing all these things and must continue to find out the secret of using each day positively. As a committed Christian it is important that my attitude to each fresh day must reflect my faith.

## UNA KROLL

Faith is a risk; it is a leap into the unknown; it is an act of conviction. Yet, in my husband, and in some other very old people I have known, I have seen a serenity in the face of doubt that speaks to me of their profound faith. Their confidence helps me to understand the great trust which Christ showed on the Cross, when in an act of total self-surrender he spoke those last words of triumphant conviction as he died, 'It is finished', and 'Father, into thy hands I commit my spirit.'

Ever since I was a small girl I have lived with people much older than I was. As I have grown older myself I have watched my husband's struggles to live a faith-centred life. I have profited from the thoughts and prayers of many enclosed nuns and monks with whom I have been closely associated. I have learnt how to die by watching older people die. I have been greatly influenced by the patient hope of very old people, who know that each moment of each day may be their last on earth, and who are nevertheless determined to enjoy and make the fullest possible use of that moment. I find in such people a kind of abandonment to divine providence, and a willingness to live or die according to God's will that teaches me more about God than anything else I can think of.

From *Growing Older* by Una Kroll (Fount 1988).


## CLARE CLUCAS

I find aspects of creation, of art and music speak to me increasingly as I get older. I listen to classical music, including sacred pieces, and I also enjoy some of the more modern songs and hymns and find they enable me to feel close to God. I have read about the life of the composer Mahler, for instance, who was searching for something, and I find this aspect of his music touches me deeply. I also find Celtic Christianity uplifting. I find God now through a quieter, more contemplative style of worship. In the congregational church decisions about worship are very much shared by members. I find there is pressure from younger people to push for noisier services. I am pleased for their energy and enthusiasm – I was like that once – but I am concerned that the need for quieter, gentler forms of worship amongst older church members can be easily overlooked.

I love the peace and beauty of creation, mountains and lakes, and the stormy sea and wind bring messages of the wonder of God the Creator. I like to learn about Christian followers, well-known and just ordinary, among the many books I read – another of my pleasures.

## THE REVD KATHLEEN LEES

The Christian Council on Ageing (CCOA) has been going now for some twelve years; it has never had a very large membership, but it is important in its very existence, because of its concern for the *spiritual* well-being of older people. As CCOA's Executive and Affiliates Secretary over several years I have found many older people are pleased to hear that there is such an organization. They may not be so keen to join, but they are glad someone cares about the spiritual alongside the physical needs. The knowledge that 'someone cares' is a reminder that God cares. It is, of course, impossible to separate the spiritual from the physical, but it is also all too easy to concentrate on the (usually easier) provision of physical needs, on the visible rather than the more hidden needs of an older person.

We who are pensioners are our own generation, a generation with specific experiences. Each one of us has at least some memories of the war, and all that the war years meant to family life. We recall a changing society, separation and bereavements, but essentially a sharing of experiences and a sense of being together. Most people who are over seventy experienced service in the armed forces, or in a reserved occupation, or had all the responsibility of home and family while others were away. For many this has surely given a special kind of strength which has taken them on through life, with a quiet, often unexpressed faith in a God who cares, who is there when we need him most. For some the horrors of war were too great to hold firm to a belief in a good God, but the passing of the years have helped. I have been told how the various fiftieth anniversary commemorations and celebrations have helped some people to talk about experiences they have not easily previously shared with others. And those with clear memories of the 1914–18 war make their own special contribution to historical and spiritual reflection.

There is another memory specific to our generation, and that is the basic spiritual education received by very nearly all of us in childhood. Most of us were 'sent' to Sunday School, while day school included 'Scripture' and religious assemblies. Many bemoan the lack of such basic education for today's children, but while I agree that there is something lacking today, I would also question whether it was all so very helpful in building a lasting spirituality for the whole of life. All too often older people seem to think they heard it all as a child, and have stayed with a childish faith (not at all the same thing as the child-like trust to which Jesus called us). Older people are often afraid to express doubt, afraid to ask questions and especially think 'the Church' is not a place for discussion.

Therefore CCOA has an important role in offering older people and those who work with them (and all of us, since we are all getting older all the time!) the opportunity for exploration, affirmation, reminiscence, and help and guidance for both private and corporate prayer and adoration. Such help and guidance is provided through the written word, the sharing of thoughts, prayers and ideas, through conferences and through contact with the individual.

I was recently involved in setting up an Arise group under the auspices of CCOA. This is a monthly gathering of neighbours and friends for coffee and plenty of noisy conversation! (In 'Arise', A is for Activity; R for Recreation; I for Inspiration; S for Service; E for Education.) Our local group has become a support group, as members face illness or bereavement, but also provides a context in which to share concerns, discuss, question and speak out, all in a very friendly environment. We have had meals together, outings and speakers and special meetings where we share hymns, readings and poems or talk about our memories of when we were younger. Often the discussion seems rather superficial; we do not readily explore deeply. But seeds are sown and we can all go away still thinking about things for ourselves. One housebound lady I collect often says: 'It makes me feel I am still part of the world!'

This article appeared first in the Newsletter of the Carers Christian Fellowship, October–December 1996.

## THE REVD DAVID WAINWRIGHT

There are many different models of spirituality in retirement, reflecting the unique needs of individual elderly people. It is also true, however, that these many accounts of spirituality in retirement show points of convergence. It is this convergence which shows that they are on the right track, for they all lead in towards the central experience of God which is the goal that we seek.

It is all too easy to put our lives into watertight compartments. We remain the same person from eight to eighty, yet we are aware of certain watersheds in life when the same person's perspective on life can change dramatically. (. . .)

This watershed is apparent on two levels. The first is the simple level of physical health. By the time of our retirement, apart from a general slowing up, the body may well be showing signs of sheer wear and tear, with bits of it beginning to show their age! (. . .)

The second level is that of a change of status. We change from being an earner to being a pensioner. Not initially with regret, for we are aware of the constraints that have been removed, of the anxieties particularly on the job front, which are no longer there. But we become increasingly aware of the way in which other people come to think of us: no longer part of the rat race, and at the same time no longer productive and of rather less importance than the rest of the working population. (. . .)

We can of course take over into our retirement a number of activities. These will largely be those in which we have a personal interest, and which could be detached from the structures of our working lives, but most other things we have to learn to relinquish. (. . .)

We can live, then, with the happinesses of our working lives, but we also have to come to terms with the things that we did not achieve, the hopes that we did not realize and the disappointments and regrets about which we can no longer do anything. (. . .)

It is when we are in this situation that a change of emphasis in our spirituality becomes relevant. Our understanding of the Christian faith does not change. All that God has done for us in Christ remains true, but when we retire one element in spirituality becomes vitally important. We need to understand a basic swing in the mode of our spirituality from *doing* to *being*. It is now not so much what we do in our activities that matters but what we are.

In fact, this has been a part of our spiritual life all along, but the pressures of work may have kept it in the background. All through our working life we have wanted to be able to be still, but the pressures of work make for an activity-oriented spirituality. If we have been wise we will see that this is punctuated by periods of retreat and recollection and the quiet of our personal daily prayer; that is the most that we can normally manage.

But now we have been relieved of those pressures and are set free simply to *be*. Just as holidays for retired people (and we will have the chance of many more of them) are not so much breaks from tiring work, but an occasion for fresh experience, we need a change of ambience, so that our spirituality will become less of a recharging of batteries and more of a realization of one who has been present to us all the time were we aware of him. We know him as the ground of our being and start to wait on him instead of being burdened by the given tasks of our paid work.

Such a spirituality is neither painless nor supine. It is an attentive waiting on God for what he will send. It is not a pursuit of activity from without, but rather one which wells up from within. There is a need in retirement to wait for things to come to you rather than to conduct frantic searches to fill a gap. It is a challenge to the 'got to keep myself busy' attitude of some retired people who see life as a gap to be filled with the treadmill of voluntary work. Rather we have been profoundly liberated for we have been freed from the super-ego-like pursuit of things to do. We may have all the sensitivities of a Christian conscience but we can learn to use them in a more relaxed way. God knows perfectly well that we are there and he will send us things to do, though they may not always be what we had expected.

What of the work that we may be called to do? It would be unprofitable to list it, because, secular or religious, it could be literally anything. What distinguishes it is that what we give is *quality time*, because what we give is what can most appropriately be given under the circumstances of our life. The former headmistress who runs a bereavement group, the housewife who runs a contemplative prayer group or the retired engineer who gives help in a drop-in centre could all be examples of appropriate responses, just as the more stereotyped demands on our time may need to prove themselves to have come from God. Retired clergy are not always available to take services, just as retired bank managers are not the inevitable choice for PCC treasurers! One lesson that we may have to learn in retirement is the ability to say no! What is important is that what we do comes from God. (. . .)

On retirement we join, as it were, the generality of the community and become immersed in it. The representative nature of what we have done before has disappeared in its more public aspects, and we are nearer than we ever were to becoming private citizens again. We have become 'unknown yet well known' and our ministry, in the widest sense, carries with it a sense of hiddenness, for it is no longer conducted from the pedestal of our active life. A clergyman is no longer the *persona* of the parish; an actor is no longer centre stage; a businessman no longer exercises commercial authority. Yet what we find ourselves doing still contains the richness of our working lives and is no less effective because it is hidden with Christ in God.

And if we have made the switch from doing to being, then our hiddenness does not signify any loss of worth or value in the sight of God. Rather such a spirituality affirms it. For the world, the 'feel-good' factor seems so essential in bolstering our egos, and giving us a sense of our own significance. Yet this is ultimately illusory and we meet people whose memory of their great days dominates their lives. Yet for Christians the truth is that we are held by God in a particular situation for his good purposes. It is this which gives perspective to our joys and to our sorrows, and helps us to realize that we have a legitimate ministry to perform even if it is a different one.

It may be felt that what has been written above has a touch too much pessimism about it. Yet it is necessary. For a spirituality to be effective, it must be laid alongside the known possibilities of human ageing. A 'golden sunset' view of retirement can only be true insofar as we take into account the human realities which accompany it. The road to the garden of resurrection has to go over the hill of Calvary.

A spirituality of ageing and retirement must be able to support us along the last stage of our human existence, when we are made increasingly aware of the diminishment and frailty of extreme old age. Sister Anke puts it in her inimitable way:

> One day my old age came into the hall . . . This old age was a very small very ancient and joyful person. She told me how she works. She said to me: I'll take away from you one thing after another, perhaps beginning with your teeth, your hair, looking young and fresh and so on. You have the choice. If you give me freewillingly what I want to have I will bring it and give it to Christ as your gift; if you refuse, I will rob you of it, because I am much stronger than you, and put it in my own pocket . . . Christ can be very creative in us when we are ready to be diminished, to let go our strength, our youth, all we are in becoming older and older. His challenges for obedience will grow – and the challenges to new creation within us.

A spirituality which is concerned with being rather than doing is a spirituality for ageing people which can withstand physical diminishment. It is not only a spirituality for early retirement but also for the time of increasing physical frailty. Bedfast or housebound, demented or diminished, we are held by God and our worth is affirmed even if to the world we seem to have so little.

This attentive waiting on God is encouraged by the great masters of the spiritual life. 'He has guided you thus far in life', writes St Francis de Sales, 'Do but hold fast to His hand and He will lead you safely through all your trials ... be at peace, then, and put aside all useless thoughts, all vain dreads and all anxious imaginings.' John Henry Newman, in a meditation, is even more definite:

> Therefore will I trust Him, wherever, whatever I am I can never be thrown away. If I am in sickness, my sickness may serve Him; in perplexity my perplexity may serve Him; if I am in sorrow my sorrow may serve Him. He does nothing in vain.

The spirituality that we have been looking at goes right along the continuum of retirement. It encompasses the crisis of first becoming retired, it makes our physical diminution ultimately irrelevant for it affirms us for who we are, held by God up to the very end of our lives.

This piece first appeared in *Plus*, the journal of the Christian Council on Ageing.

---

## Life's Journey

When we start out on our journey
with Jesus as our guide
We need a place to come apart
We need a place to hide

So young in Christ so much to learn
And so much work to do
Watching out for Satan's darts
While staying strong and true

But then as we're getting older
And feeling more secure
Then we get a little bolder
So our steps become more sure

But when we reach our journey's end
And feeling old and frail
With Jesus still close by our side
We'll enter through the vale

To see our blessed Saviour's face
To know of his great love
When we this earthly race have run
We'll dwell with him above
                                    Betty Maclean


## PROFESSOR BARONESS McFARLANE OF LLANDAFF

My life started in a Christian home. Both my father and mother were committed Christians and looking back I see that I imbibed my faith almost along with my mother's milk. My mother was a warm, and welcoming person. My earliest memories are of being nursed in her arms as she sang some of the old Sankey Moody and Fanny Crosbie hymns. The words of many of them still come back to me in unexpected moments. One of them she sang was,

> In the shadow of His wings
> There is rest, sweet rest.

I used to join in and sing

> In the shadow of his swings!

An older friend met me recently and asked, 'Are you still living in the shadow of his swings?' I could say, 'Yes, I am' and I recognize the great sense of security that has given me all my life!

By contrast my father, a doctor, was more intellectual in his approach to faith. He learned Greek and Hebrew so that he could understand the Bible to better advantage. His biblical teaching was vivid and memorable. I recognize strands of the faith of both of my parents in myself; the simplicity of faith and the need to worship with all my mind.

There is no doubt that, as retirement progresses, certain powers decrease. As I watch my friends I find this is variable for different people. After eight years of retirement, I have a far less retentive memory. I used to read widely and be able to recall and give references to my students with little effort. I no longer have that ability. I used to travel extensively to the House of Lords and give lectures in various parts of the country and the world. I now find travelling from Manchester to London and back in the same day tiring.

If there are some losses, there are great gains. A close and extensive family is a great asset. For my seventieth birthday we had one family party in England and one in Canada and on the day itself I held an open house for my church family. Those three events made me feel that I was cocooned in the love of so many people and that our basic sharing was of the love of God. So the focus of my identity has shifted from who I am as a professional person, innovative and expressing my faith through a caring profession, to someone who is loved supremely by God and his people, able to let go some of the things that once were important and to stretch out to a future of identity with him.

My life is not without peaks and troughs and I struggle with my own spirituality in the process of ageing. At a rational level, I see that the vocation I now have and the role I occupy may have to change. For how long can one continue to teach and preach? For how long can one be an effective member of the House of Lords? For how long can one be physically active? My mother lived to 108 and I saw various stages to her ageing. Sometimes I wonder, as time goes on and the physical and mental abilities decrease, if I will be called to what perhaps may be the most important role in my life, a life of prayer. The first definition of the word 'retire' given in my dictionary is 'withdraw, go away, retreat, seek seclusion or shelter, recede, go to bed'. All that sounds rather negative! But I like to think that the human body and mind in their greatest deterioration are still of value. I used to sit beside my mother when there was no apparent response and think, 'That poor old body is still a temple of the Holy Spirit.' There is a significance and value to life in all its stages and perhaps we place too great an emphasis on achievement rather than being.

### MARY JORDAN

I have been widowed twice, the first time when I was relatively young. The second time I was quite a bit older and the circumstances were totally different. It was a tragic time for myself and for my family, and to some extent I felt cut off from normality, but God speaks in different ways and so what came to me may not be what he gives to all. The God I discovered in the Bible at that time is described in Isaiah:

'Do not be afraid; you will not suffer shame.
Do not fear disgrace; you will not be humiliated.
You will forget the shame of your youth
and remember no more the reproach of your
    widowhood.
For your Maker is your husband –
the Lord Almighty is his name –
the Holy One of Israel is your Redeemer;
he is called the God of all the earth.
The Lord will call you back
as if you were a wife deserted and distressed in spirit –
a wife who married young,
only to be rejected,' says your God.

'For a brief moment I abandoned you,
but with deep compassion I will bring you back.
In a surge of anger
I hid my face from you for a moment,
but with everlasting kindness
I will have compassion on you,'
says the Lord your Redeemer. (Isaiah 54.4-8)

I have these verses circled in my Bible. I cannot always live up to these promises but knowing he will and does is blessing in itself. In periods of loneliness, tiredness and sickness it is good to know that the Lord is still there giving guidance and blessing, and that he will answer if I ask. Out of my experiences, I wrote the following poem:

### Our Father God, Forever Near

Our Father God, forever near,
In times of trouble, calm our fear,
Today and yesterday the same,
Your saving grace, through Christ, who came.

Restrain our wills, dear Lord we pray,
That we may walk your perfect way,
Our thoughts and minds and wills control,
Our lips to utter words made whole.

O Holy Spirit, none can flee,
May you our strength and comfort be.
We reign triumphant when we seek
The victory yours, our work complete.

You give to all who wait your word
Your strength in weakness, precious Lord,
That we may all your will obey,
Keep walking in your perfect way.

We praise our Father God today,
Our Saviour is our chosen way,
The Holy Spirit, he our guide,
These Three are One and by our side.

# 8

# Looking Ahead

Young people conduct their lives as if the future stretches ahead of them without end, leaving unlimited time in which to accomplish goals and fulfil dreams. Death is a remote speck on the horizon, a distant eventuality which they are reluctant to discuss.

Older people, on the other hand, can escape thoughts of death for only so long. Eventually its reality is impressed upon them through the loss of loved ones. In time older people usually achieve a greater level of acceptance than younger people are able to cultivate. They develop a more honest and balanced approach to death and most can discuss it frankly. Sadly their attempts to talk openly about it are often suppressed by the younger people around them: 'Don't be morbid, Gran.'

The hospice movement has done much to help us face death with equanimity. It used to be a doctor's prerogative to conceal from a patient the facts about terminal illness. The hospice movement encourages professionals and relatives alike to see that allowing a dying person to recognize what is happening can give them permission to face up to its implications and put their affairs in order.

We all harbour fears about death, whatever our age. As several contributors to this book admit, the fear is often over the process of dying itself, and the possibility of protracted pain or loss of dignity and self-control. For others, Christians included, the dread has more to do with what will occur after death, and with images of God's judgement.

The Christian faith offers great comfort to those who fear the transition from this world to the next. We learn in Scripture that our new life has already begun, but that it will reach its fulfilment only when we die. There is continuity here for the Christian. For those who are facing death it helps to see their own passing not as the experience of an isolated individual, but in the context of their place in the wider world. The work they have begun is not ending. Its effects will live on and give benefit to those who are still living. Tasks they consider important can be handed on to the next generation. In dying older people can look back and rejoice over the faithfulness of God throughout their lives.

Because of the proximity of death, older people are often receptive to spiritual things and respond with joy to the good news about saving grace. Some of the uncertainty and fearfulness they feel over death is then replaced by a peaceful assurance of God's love and of the welcome with which he awaits their arrival.

## MARGARET WILLIAMS

### On Mount Tabor

Old age, for this old lady at least, has proved to be Mount Tabor. It has taken ninety years for us, the Lord and I, to climb this far, but now we are sitting down at last, by ourselves, very near the top. The view is glorious, a whole lifetime of the Lord's goodness, seen in perspective. We have come to this high place to pray together; the world is sorely in need of prayer.

And now he is showing me something of what he really is; he has become transfigured before me. He is wearing his earthly garments. His face is radiant; his eyes are fixed on me as though I mattered. He is speaking to his Father who, unseen in a bright cloud,

calls him 'beloved Son'. Is the bright cloud the Holy
Spirit? Life has become trinitarian of late.

Two friends have suddenly joined us: Madeleine
Sophie and Philippine. That shows that heaven is not
very far away. He tells me not to be afraid, and touches
me. It is good to be here, but he will not let me pitch
a tent. We must wait under the stars for a time, until
he tells us to stand up and set off for the last short
climb to the door of home. It has begun to open.

> From *On the Way Home: Reflections for Old Age*, ed.
> Frances Makower  and Joan Faber
> (Darton, Longman and Todd 1994).


## CLARE CLUCAS

I cannot imagine heaven. Perhaps arriving there resembles
a recent experience I had of waking from a general anaes-
thetic. From complete oblivion I passed to light and an
awareness of people around caring for me. I believe that 'in
my Father's house are many mansions' and know that I can
trust these words of promise because Jesus spoke them.

Like many people I hope for a quick and painless death
and, perhaps more than anything, I would like to remain
in possession of my mental faculties, as did my parents and
members of my wider family. I would hate to be a trouble
to my children and I tell them that, if I reach the state of
health of another elderly relative of ours, they must put me
in a home!


## LORD COGGAN

Retirement is, from one point of view, a bereavement. If
one has enjoyed work and been devoted to it, its ending is
inevitably a loss. A friend of mine said to me at the time
of the death of her husband: 'On the day of his retirement
[that was thirteen years previously] he died.' That is the
wrong way to regard retirement, so negative as to lead to
depression if not to bitterness. Retirement need not – should

not – be regarded so negatively, for it can, and often does, open up new possibilities of development, of fulfilment, and of usefulness. There are fresh vistas awaiting exploration.

I realize that I have been immensely fortunate in the years since I retired in 1980. I have a loving family and a life-partner beyond all praise. I have had – and still have – more than enough work to do. I have a mind which, though it plays tricks on me with increasing frequency, still functions and enables me to write and speak, to enjoy people and music and art and books. The oncoming of old age has been gradual and for that I thank God constantly. Many of my friends of a similar age have not been so fortunate.

Sorrows and difficulties? Of course. The death of so many relatives and friends; decreasing vigour and increasing creaks of body and mind; limitations; coming to terms with the insistent 'why?' which prefaces so many issues which hitherto could be brushed aside or ignored, and being content with having no answers to persistent questions . . . One could go on. But thankfulness to God for his sheer goodness and graciousness brings a sunshine which penetrates the shadows. And hope – well, I wrote a book about it five years ago [*God of Hope* (HarperCollins 1991)] – perhaps it means more, now that time will soon give place to eternity and we shall 'be like him, for we shall see him as he is'.

The passing of the years gives a sense of proportion denied to us in our earlier decades. Some issues which then seemed to us of great importance, now appear to have shrunk – why did we fuss about such trivialities? They have receded as other matters of more abiding significance have taken their place. A sense of proportion brings peace.

Regrets? Of course. Sins of commission, sins of omission, opportunities un-seized or ill-used; so many gifts from God not made the most of . . . Again, one could go on. But to stay too long in the dark world of retrospect and regret is unhealthy. 'There is forgiveness with thee.' And forgiveness, surely, is the greatest of God's gifts and is to be received with open hands. The only thing to do with our sins, our

lost opportunities, is to leave them at the foot of Christ's
cross:

> At thy feet I lay them,
> And I leave them there.

Only recently I came across these lines of Studdert Kennedy.
In offering to God 'this writing of the years', he said:

> I can but hand it in, and hope
> that thy great mind, which reads
> the writings of so many lives,
> will understand this scrawl
> and what it strives
> to say – but leaves unsaid.

Studdert Kennedy knew a thing or two about humankind
and life and death – and God!

In October 1995 I had the privilege of preaching in
Westminster Abbey at a service to mark the United Nations
International Day for Elderly People. I began my sermon
thus:

The story is told of an early British king, a pagan, who
was puzzled about the meaning of life as he experienced
it. To him it seemed to lack all meaning. It was, he said,
like the passage of a bird flying out of the darkness
through a well-lit hall and flying out again into the dark
– and that was that. This was the concept of a pagan
king. It is the very antithesis of what Christians believe.
It is said of Jesus Christ that he knew that 'he came
from God and that he was going back to God.' Between
those two poles his life was lived. He came from God;
therefore God had a purpose which he must fulfil. He
was going back to God: therefore life was moving towards
a goal, a climax . . . Life seen like that has a dignity and
a significance all its own.

I would want to add: 'Death has a glory all its own.'

'Going back to God' – isn't that the right way to envisage death? Back to the God who loves us with a love more pure and intense than any human love we have experienced; back to the God who waits to welcome us home, as he has welcomed home our relatives and friends in Christ who have died before us. With them we are 'knit together into one communion and fellowship', and 'death itself cannot unbind [our] happy brotherhood'.

It is natural – and understandable – that we should anticipate with distaste the process of passing from this life to that, if that process is long and continued and distressing. We can only pray that we may be given the grace of being good recipients at the hands of those who are there to help us. No: there is more to it than that. There is a confidence given to the Christian disciple to which John Henry Newman gave apt expression when he wrote:

> So long thy power hath blest me, sure it still
> will lead me on,
> o'er moor and fen, o'er crag and torrent, till
> the night is gone,
> and with the morn those angel faces smile
> which I have loved long since, and lost awhile.

With that confidence we 'fearful saints' may 'fresh courage take'.

---

### Autumn

*After a sharp frost, on a windless morning, I*
*watched leaves falling . . .*

The frost has made the leaves
Lose their grip. Like pattering rain,
They fall, returning to earth.

Might death be like that,
A gentle falling to the dust
From which I came?

Must I go raging into that
Dark night? Could I not,
As the sharp frost of age
Begins to chill,
Simply let go?

Ann Lewin

## BISHOP LESSLIE NEWBIGIN

As I look forward, I find my inspiration in Philippians 3 where Paul describes his own attitude to the past and to the future. I find myself compelled by this vision of the athlete who is determined to continue the race until it is finished and who looks with eager longing towards the goal. And of course, that goal is not just something for myself and my loved ones but is the consummation of all things in which above all our Lord Jesus Christ will see the travail of his soul and be satisfied. Like the mountaineers Mallory and Irvine on Everest, who were last seen 'going strong for the top', I would hope and pray that I might continue pressing forward in the sure hope of the kingdom which is prepared for us.

## REG WYATT

I am saved. The Lord is preparing a place for me in Heaven. I shall see him there. It will be a place without tears, strife or pain. This summarizes my Christian hope for the future.

Having said that, I'm not one for spending time attempting to visualize what heaven will be like; I will know when I get there. My effort now must be in doing my best to live according to God's will and purpose. A place in heaven can be viewed as a reward, but I regard it essentially as being wholly a gift of God's grace. I have not specifically prepared to meet death or terminal illness, apart from the one practicality of making a will, I suppose because neither seems imminent. I do not fear death in the sense of extinction, for I have a future beyond death. I do, however, feel uncomfortable about the prospect of prolonged illness, severe pain or physical disablement. I hope my trust in God will enable me, in his strength, to cope with these things if they come. It certainly did two years ago when I was diagnosed as having prostate cancer, which, praise God, has been cured.

As to assessing what I will leave behind after death, I do not know what legacy of accomplishments will remain. Somehow, I think I shall leave others to make the assessment, because they can do so dispassionately. I think I would be content to say that I have tried hard and done my best most of the time. If others could agree with that, I shall be satisfied. One thing I would not like, although I shall not be in a position to hear what is said, is a eulogy at my funeral, because I know that I have as many faults as virtues.

---

From sudden death,
Good Lord, deliver us.

But death is always sudden,
Slipping between one moment
And eternity. We can't escape.
Indeed, it's what I hope for.
Not for me painful diminishment
Of long, slow dying: that's
Much more to be feared.

The trouble is, that
When death suddenly
Catches our breath,
We leave behind loose ends,
Relationships at odds,
Or words unsaid:
Fuel for guilt for those

Surviving, quite apart
From any personal
Dissatisfaction.

Perhaps our prayer should be
For more awareness;
Not preoccupation
With our mortal end,
But aliveness to
This moment's possibilities.
It may just be our last.

*For* sudden death,
Good Lord, prepare us.

Ann Lewin

## LORD SOPER

Looking back over a very long life I am astonished at the comparative indifference of my earlier years to the prospect of life after death. I professed it publicly as a Methodist preacher, but it seemed such a long way off that for me it was relatively unimportant.

It was Dr Johnson who said, 'A sentence of death marvellously concentrates the mind.' Now it is unquestionable that we are all under such a sentence from the day we were born, but as far as I can remember the thought of the inevitable conclusion to my life hardly entered my head for decades, let alone concentrated my attention. I took immortality for granted until the proximity of death was impressed upon me by the death of relatives, or the casualties of war. Even then the thought could be shrugged off – but not as the past lengthens and the future shortens.

Now I am an old man, and to put it simply, death is a very 'live' issue, and words like heaven and hell have an unavoidable immediacy. In fact, I am convinced that to realize that our human experience on this planet is not the sum total of reality has become an absolute requirement.

All our aspirations as to the quality of life after death, all our anticipation that human relationships will be restored after being severed on earth, all questions about what it will be like for the good and the bad – all this ultimately depends on whether heaven is a 'must or a myth'.

I am now satisfied that if there is any truth anywhere, it can only be credible if there is an optimistic future beyond the grave. So as I peer into the future with an added urgency, I find my comfort not in any precise plan of eternity, but in the confidence that the God of creation and of providence revealed by Jesus will be 'there', just as I believe he is 'here', and I shall be a member of his family. I will be content with that. In other words, there is a concentration of mind which results from the recognition of death. To direct that concentration to God, and to Jesus as his human photograph, rather than to the conditions of the next world, is the secret of tranquility and contentment.

I believe that 'God is love' demands a realm of experience where fulfilment of his loving purpose can happen – and it cannot fully happen in the world of time and space and matter. I can and ought to begin that pilgrimage, here and now, to his kingdom, but I need that eternal world so that as I start out, like Christian in *The Pilgrim's Progress*, I cannot only find the wages of going on from day to day, but can catch the sound of the trumpets that will sound for me on the other side. The more I think about the prospect of death, the more it appears as a gateway rather than a terminus. But if it leads to a realm beyond time and space I shall waste no time in trying to picture it, and no space in trying to put it into words. What I can do is to think more deeply about the kind of God who is the source of all being and whose nature I see in Jesus. The future is in his hands and there I can safely leave it.

Here I must add a strong note of caution. In the foregoing I have assumed that I am going to heaven, but I am not at all sure about that. I must make certain that I do not go to the other place. I have a responsibility now to order my life in the best way I can, by the grace of God. Therefore my preoccupation must be with the moral and spiritual requirements which, if obeyed, will enable me to dwell in the house of the Lord forever. What can turn that obligation into good news is that Jesus is for me the way into that house, the truth about its many rooms, and the life of that household forever.

I believe in hell, both here and hereafter. Hell is the absence of the love of God; it is the deliberate or actual death of hope and faith in the ultimate reality of goodness. There are many people who know about that hell down here, and I see no reason to suppose that at the point of death that process will stop. I think for them it will probably go on in the direction in which it has been going. I believe that what I begin on this planet will not be cut short by death, but can be continued and enlarged.

Similarly with relationships. We already have experiences on this planet of being together in unity. I belong to a family and the family belongs to me. We do not all agree but we belong, and this gives the sense of identity. Separation is the greatest of evils and the greatest of sorrows. To belong – to be associated with and identified with other human beings – that must prevail in heaven, or I do not want to go there.

Incidentally, the next stage of human existence may be elsewhere in this amazing universe, but I have better things to do than to idle away the hours in such a reverie. So much of the future is a 'cloud of unknowing' but it need not obscure the light of faith which sings, 'I'll praise him for all that is past and trust him for all that's to come.'

Meanwhile I have no intention of waiting beside the 'silent sea' to hear the 'muffled oar'. Alongside the hope of the future is the fact that human beings do make their own history, and today's history is yesterday's choice. So looking forward may be a leap in the dark, but the leap as it is taken enlightens that darkness. This surely is the underlying message of Jesus, as set forth in the Sermon on the Mount. Obedience today is the key to well-being tomorrow. To be pacific, humble, pure in heart, avid for goodness and ready to pay its price – these are the articles of obedience which govern the future. Only by such obedience on my part do I put the future into God's hands where alone it will be safe and beneficent.

Nevertheless, the question will nag at my mind. Is the above the indulgence of a myth rather than the practice of an adventure? Is our contemplation of the future fundamentally subjective rather than objective? I must choose as an experiment, so that the practice of hope of eternity is the very road to that eternity, requiring a conversion of my mind and heart. This is the ultimate meaning of the conversion experience. By grace I am saved, through faith, and that is the gift of God, and if I ask for it he will not say me nay.

## PAUL TOURNIER

What embarrasses me is that I cannot repeat what I hear so often, and what is perhaps expected of me, that the meaning of my old age is to prepare me for death and for meeting God, to detach me from the things of the world in order to attach me to those of heaven. I doubt if I should ever be ready, especially if I concerned myself henceforth only with preparing myself for it. Death will come for me just as I am, and what happens to me will depend exclusively, as it will for all other men, my brethren, on God's mercy, and not on my preparation, however sincere it may be.

In my view it is the whole of life which is a preparation for death, and I do not see how I can prepare myself any differently today than at any other time. Death is not a project, and it is not my reality. What concerns me is my life now, and to seek the will of God for me today, for the meaning of life seems to me to be always the same, from one end to the other – to allow oneself to be led by God. Detach myself from the world? That would be to run away from my own reality . . . .

A sentence from St Paul will help me to define my thought. It is well-known: 'Though this outer man of ours may be falling into decay, the inner man is renewed day by day' (1 Corinthians 4.16).

From *Learning to Grow Old* by Paul Tournier
(English tr., SCM Press 1972).

## HARRY GOOCH

Notwithstanding the possibility of death through accident or terminal illness, which can assail us at any time in our lives, the inevitable end to this life looms nearer and more clearly as we reach three score years and ten.

I have found in my Christian life that however great our gift of faith (and it is a gift), the need for reassurance often grows apace as we begin to slow down with advancing years. To step from this known world, with all its complexities of joys and sorrows, into a world which through faith is much more to be desired, is not easy. The one is a known fact, the other a hopeful fact through faith.

Many of my Christian friends over the years who have shown love and understanding to those facing crises in their lives, spreading hope and reassurance, have found that they too needed the same love and reassurance when facing similar situations. The young Christian may depend on the 'wisdom' of the old, but the old Christian needs the 'lively assurance' of the young.

Some years ago I lost, through industrial injury, a dear Christian friend, and the need for reassurance flooded into my consciousness. I had a vivid dream which did not die when I woke, but stayed with me in clear detail. I later used this dream in a poem. In it there is doubt, reassurance, hope and victory:

## My Dream

I laughed, sun-drenched in summer's radiance;
I wandered, knee-deep in flowered profusion;
I sang, enraptured, the ephemeral songs of earth.

I met a strange and awesome building;
I saw a dark and windowless room;
I heard a voice utter words of warning;
I felt oppressed by gathering gloom.

'Do not put foot inside this door
Unless you can stand the stench of death!'

I turned aside, I sang no more;
I dared not step inside that door.

The sun had set, the flowers withered,
No longer warmed by summer air;
I shivered, chilled; I stood alone,
Those who had walked with me had gone.

I heard an urgent unseen voice;
I swung around to learn its source;
He stood, from head to foot, a King!
Upon his head a crown of gold;
His hair like wool or driven snow;
His eyes like flames of fire;
His hands an orb and sceptre held.

'I have conquered death!' he cried,
'I am the beginning and the end of time;
Fear not to take that final earthbound step
Into my eternity!'

I felt new life flow in my veins;
I sang again, but not the songs of earth;
I sang the eternal hymns of heaven!

I turned and stepped into that door;
Head held high, I walked in fear no more.

There bathed in his redeeming light,
I met my God!

# Further Reading

J. Burton-Jones, *From Generation to Generation: Towards a Christian Understanding of the Role and Care of Older People* (Jubilee Centre Publications 1990).

O. Butler and A. Orbach, *Being Your Age: Pastoral Care for Older People* (SPCK 1993).

E. Church, *For Ever Jubilant: The Adventure of Ageing*, available from E. Church, 52 Mill Road, Salisbury, Wiltshire SP2 7RZ, price £2.80 (proceeds to Salisbury Diocesan Sudan Medical Link).

A. Creber, *New Approaches to Ministry with Older People* (Grove Books 1990).

R. Davis, *My Journey into Alzheimer's Disease: Helpful Insights for Family and Friends* (Tyndale House 1989).

U. Kroll, *Growing Older* (Fount Paperbacks 1988).

F. Makower and J. Faber (eds), *On the Way Home: Reflections for Old Age* (Darton, Longman and Todd 1994).

E. Midwinter, *The British Gas Report on Attitudes to Ageing 1991* (British Gas 1991).

H. J. M. Nouwen and Walter J. Gaffney, *Aging: The Fulfillment of Life* (Doubleday 1976).

P. Tournier, *Learning to Grow Old* (English tr., SCM 1972).